Menopause Action Plan

*Your Essential Guide
to Heal Your Hypothalamus
and Thrive during the Change of Life*

Deborah Maragopoulos FNP

Genesis Health Products, Inc Ojai, California

Copyright © 2021 by Deborah Maragopoulos FNP

All rights reserved. No part of this book may be reproduced in any manner without written permission except for quotations embodied in critical articles and reviews. For additional information contact

Genesis Health Products, Inc
222 Sierra Road
Ojai, CA 93023

A publication of Genesis Health Products, Inc

Print ISBN: 978-1-940112-04-6

Ebook ISBN: 978-1-940112-05-3

Cover art: The Change by Ann Marie Simon

Get your fillable Menopause Action Plan here: GenesisGold.com/MAP

*For my mother,
Maria Ann Diodato,
who taught me that to heal a woman,
heals her family, her community, the world*

Acknowledgments

I am so very grateful for all the assistance I received while writing this book. MAP has definitely been a labor of love. My own long journey through menopause, as well as my experience helping thousands of women navigate the change of life, have provided the impetus to write this book, but there have also been so many people who have helped throughout the process.

First and foremost, my husband, who lovingly supports me in everything I do, encouraged me to complete this book and supported me through the emotional process that is inherent in publishing. I'd like to thank my team who have been fantastic at helping get this project from conception to launch, particularly my operations manager, Amber Kinney and her team, and my faithful assistant, Gabriela Tapia.

I'd like to thank my book coach, Mary Anne Radmacher, for supporting my idea of writing this revolutionary book and helping me find the contacts necessary to get the book in print. I'd like to thank my editor, Kathleen Everett RN, and my copy editor, Mackenzie Roark, for doing a great job of helping me make all the medical terminology understandable.

Last but not least, I would like to thank all of the women who participated in my debut Menopause Action Plan workshop. I'm so thankful for these women who were attentive as I presented the material, asked provocative questions, shared stories of creating their own successful Menopause Action Plans, and encouraged me to get this book out there.

Contents

Introduction ... ix

Part One
You are Here
1. The Change of Life Starts Here ... 3
2. Where are You in the Change? ... 12

Part Two
Learning the Lay of the Land
3. What Happens in the Change? ... 31
4. The Most Common Symptoms ... 39
5. Lesser Known Symptoms ... 50
6. Your Risk Factors ... 70

Part Three
Connecting the Dots
7. The Hypothalamic Connection ... 93
8. The Gifts of Menopause ... 113

Part Four
Choosing Your Vehicle
9. Hormone Replacement Therapy ... 139
10. Alternative Therapies ... 168

Part Five
Packing for the Trip
11. Pillars of Healing ... 195
12. Empowered Menopause ... 221
13. Tools to Thrive ... 243

APPENDIX

References 249

About the Author 273

Introduction

I create my flow. You create your flow. And that flow is your physical health, your vitality, your relationships. It's the connections you have with the earth, with the people around you, with everything. You're in control of that flow. In order to stay in control, you need to be as educated as possible about what's happening in your body, and how it's affecting your mind, your relationships, and all of your connections.

I see life as a kind of trilogy, with maidenhood being the first book. Youth is the time when we discover who we are. Motherhood is the second book. You don't have to be a mother to experience the joy of creation; whether it be your work or your hobbies, as a woman, your adult years are a highly creative time. And this transition called the *change of life* delivers us into our cronehood, a time to share our wisdom. The change begins the third book of our life. And as exciting as the story may have been so far, it's going to get even more exciting.

When you go through the change of life, everything changes. It's not just the physical symptoms you're feeling. The change affects how you think, how you experience your emotions, and it affects everyone around you. As a woman, you know intimately how much you are affected by other people's energy and their hormones.

Have you ever worked or lived with a group of other women and you all started menstruating together? That's the communal effect of hormones, pheromones, and vibration. It's part of our survival technique that we resonate with one another.

When we get out of balance hormonally, it affects everyone around us, whether we like it or not, and whether we're aware of it or not. Because of this, we have to be prepared for the change, because menopause is inevitable.

When you were in high school, you probably took a health class. Oftentimes, the boys and girls were separated, so the teacher could discuss the changes your body would be going through, which would be spurred by your hormones. This book was designed to prepare you mentally, if not emotionally, for adolescence.

If you have children, you may have begun to prepare them for the changes that puberty brings long before high school health class. I started talking to my kids early about what to expect. I wanted them to have as much education as possible about how their bodies work, and all the changes – physical, mental, emotional and spiritual – they might experience so they would be prepared.

I talk to my young female patients about the change long before it's going to happen so they can be prepared to make good decisions before they have to face menopause. If a patient is already on the hormonal rollercoaster of menopause, we deal with symptoms and make a plan for her future to ensure she lives her best life. And if they're already postmenopausal, I help my patients make the best decisions about their health and wellbeing so they can truly enjoy the last book of their life.

I help all my female patients create a MAP to best navigate the change.

And that's what I want to do for you. I want to help you create a MAP – your personal Menopause Action Plan.

If you're premenopausal, let's get you prepared for the change. If you're perimenopausal, let's help you hang in there as you get through menopause. If you're facing menopause right now, let's support you through the process. And if you're postmenopausal, you can have a plan to thrive instead of just survive the rest of your life, and take the right steps to avoid chronic illnesses.

I'm going to address not just the physicality of your hormones, but also their vibration. I envision your Menopause Action Plan as a rainbow path to an empowered menopause. Everything in your body is connected. Your endocrine glands correspond to chakras. From your red root survival chakra all the way up to your purple crown chakra of divine connection, you become the queen of your life.

This is a wondrous opportunity to make a significant shift, and start a brand new book in your life.

My wish for you is that you experience a graceful change and empowered menopause. I invite you to not merely survive, but to thrive in the final book of your life!

You're going to have questions.

I plan to cover everything possible about the change and how to create your own Menopause Action Plan. You might have more questions. And, frankly, there's research being done all the time that supports the reported experience of women undergoing the change. So I have a Menopause Action Plan workshop for your ongoing support that you'll get special access to by reading this book.

This book is divided into five sections:

In Part 1, you're going to discover exactly where you are in the change, which phase you're in, how your shifting hormones are affecting that phase, and what to look forward to. Yes, *look forward to*, not to regret, not to be afraid of.

In Part 2, you're going to learn how your declining sex hormones are affecting the most common symptoms in menopause. Also included are the lesser known symptoms of the change including everything that affects your nervous system, your dermatological system (your skin, hair, nails), your muscles and skeleton, your connective tissues, your immune system, and your gastrointestinal system. Essentially, you'll quickly learn that your hormones affect everything. A lot of women have uncommon symptoms, and they don't realize it's menopause. Additionally, a lot of healthcare providers are unaware that menopause can cause all these symptoms.

Then we will explore your risk factors, including your genetics, your family history, your personal history – many more questions than you'll be asked by your healthcare provider. All of these factors are super important when trying to make the best decisions for yourself around how to deal with the symptoms of the change and live your best life.

In Part 3, I'm going to cover all your connections. Physically, via your hypothalamus – the master controller of all your hormones – and how the change affects your other hormones and the rest of your body. Then, we're going to go over your psychospiritual connections, how your menopause mindset affects your experience. And we're going to explore the gifts of menopause. Yes, there are gifts. And the more that you can look forward to and recognize those gifts, the more likely they're going to serve you well going through this change.

In Part 4, I'll cover all your treatment options. First, hormone replacement therapy, including bioidenticals, and all the different delivery systems, as well as their pros and cons. We will also discuss your other hormones besides estrogen, progesterone, and testosterone, including DHEA, thyroid hormone, growth hormone, and all the other hormones that may be affected by the change. I will cover some of the options that you can use, as well as alternative and natural treatments including supplementation, homeopathy, essential oils, and energy treatments, like acupuncture and body work.

In Part 5, I'm going to give you my recommendations. I'll cover lifestyle, diet, exercise, sleep, and stress reduction. And then we'll talk about the next step in your empowered menopause, including what you need from your healthcare provider to ensure that everything is working in your favor so that this can become your time to thrive.

By the end of this book, you're going to be so educated and empowered that you will be able to confidently bring your personalized MAP to your healthcare provider and say, "This is my Menopause Action Plan, and this is what I need."

What is a Menopause Action Plan?

You're reading this book because you're interested in being as informed as possible and having a plan by which to go through the change, right? Just like if you were starting a business, you would write a plan that includes your goals and what you would need. A business plan helps you birth your business. Similarly, I see a Menopause Action Plan just like a birth plan.

If you had children, you may have developed your own birth plan. The idea of a birth plan started in the '70s, and was initiated by midwives and doulas who informed women that they have more choices than getting sedated to give birth. Pregnant women became empowered to create their own birth plans. Birth plans became so popular that they shifted obstetrics. Doctors and hospitals began incorporating women's birth plans into pregnancy care, as well as labor and delivery.

This is what I want for you. Your own personal Menopause Action Plan to empower you to navigate the change in the best way to serve you. These are **your** decisions; it's not up to your healthcare provider. Yet, how do you get their guidance? How do you get them to prescribe what you need, or do the diagnostic testing you need? Empowerment to get what you need is a big part of your Menopause Action Plan.

But first, you need to have a better understanding of what you need. I do not want you going to your health care provider at 45 with a breast lump and symptoms of perimenopause, not knowing your choices for treatment. I want you to be prepared. Even if you're in your 70s, you still have a good 20, 30, 40 years to live, and I want you to be prepared for the years ahead, so you're as healthy and vital as possible.

Your Menopause Action Plan is not only about planning for your future. It's about taking actions *now* so that you're living your best life.

Part One

You are Here

Chapter 1

The Change of Life Starts Here

I know this sounds crazy, but I was one of those strange women who actually looked forward to menopause. So many women are afraid of aging, losing their vitality, their fertility. They watch as the older women around them lose their positions in the workplace. They dread not feeling as sexy or beautiful as they used to, investing in wrinkle creams, and watching their figures shift from youthful slenderness to the thickening of middle-age.

I didn't expect that was going to happen to me. Of course, I knew I would age like everyone, but truthfully, it's been a rather graceful transition. I believe that's because I was prepared for the change.

As an intuitive integrative nurse practitioner, I've been taking care of women going through the change since 1987. Back then, I felt too young to even consider my own eventual menopause, but I noticed something about these women. When their hormones were out of balance, they shifted into a different state of mind. They became more empowered than they had been as younger women. They were more sure of themselves. They seemed to have a wisdom about them that I just couldn't grasp when I was in my 20s and 30s, but definitely appreciated.

They seemed to be happier in the moment. Certainly more joyous than I was in the moment. It's not that they didn't have stressors. It's not that they weren't challenged by life – by working full time, while taking care of households, pets, children, aging parents, and their own symptoms. Yet, they seemed to be open to new possibilities, as if they were starting a new chapter in their lives. So I started to look forward to that chapter in my own life, thinking that going through menopause was going to shift everything.

In 2003, I wrote my first book and began the journey of rediscovering my femininity, the sacredness of being a woman. It was a long journey, a tough journey, an empowering journey.

By 2007, my novel *LoveDance*® was published, and I got invited to speak to women's groups. One was the grandmother's council here in my hometown of Ojai, California.

I was so impressed by these women. This circle of postmenopausal women offered genuine heartfelt blessings to others – younger women, men, children – whoever was in need. It stirred in me a remembrance of a time when women in their crone years were revered. These grandmothers were so full of wisdom and light that I couldn't wait to be in that stage of life so that I could join the circle.

So I spent my 40s looking forward to the change, hoping that I too would be able to share my wisdom with others. Hoping that somehow, all the stories that I lived as a younger woman would finally come together, and I would be able to offer them up to women of all ages, but particularly to those going through the change. I was ready to finally be able to show them that this transition is not the end of the good parts of their life, but the beginning of the best part of their life.

And that is exactly what I hope for you. That you find hope in reading this book. That you walk away feeling prepared for the best part of your life.

I will say upfront that we're going to start with the tough stuff – the annoying uncomfortable symptoms. It's going to seem overwhelming, but I want you to understand what's happening in your body, and what kind of shifts might be happening in your mind, even in your soul. I want you to appreciate that you're going to resonate at a much higher vibration than ever before. And that you too will experience the joy of menopause.

The change can be a scary thing. All these symptoms are not fun to look forward to. Yet, just as puberty happens to everyone, every woman goes through the change. It's going to happen sooner or later, and the best way to prepare for the change and handle all these menopausal symptoms is to develop a plan – your own Menopause Action Plan – so you can deal with the symptoms, prevent complications, and live your best life.

First, you need to know where you are in the change.

Let's start with what the change looks like, in order to pinpoint where you might be. We'll also talk about your sex hormones so you understand a little bit more about what's happening.

The change is a decline in your sex hormones: estrogen, progesterone, and testosterone. However, it doesn't happen all at once. Most women do not go from 28-day regular cycles from the time of their first period until they're 50 years old, and then, at the age of 51 - boom! - their periods stop. That is very, very rare. Most women experience a slow decline of their sex hormones. Meaning that up to 15 years before they have their last period, they start to notice a decline. Now, most of my patients are incredibly intuitive and in touch with their bodies, and notice that something's off, or they wouldn't come to see me in the first place.

The majority of women may not be paying attention to what's happening in their body, or more likely, no one is paying attention to their complaints. They have to wait until something breaks to know for sure that something's off. They have to get a major disease before they consider, *maybe this is my hormones?*

Honestly, when you start having palpitations and you go to a cardiologist, they're not going to think your hormones are to blame. When you go see your therapist because you're super depressed or anxious, she's not going to suspect that it's your hormones that are causing your mood issues.

When your cholesterol starts rising, and your family doctor says, "Hey, you need to start taking a statin," he's not going to recognize that it's your hormones causing a rise in your cholesterol.

It's your declining hormones that cause most of these issues. We need to pay attention to what our hormones are, and why they're good for us. Yes, *good for us*. Some women are afraid of hormones because they believe that hormones cause cancer, or that hormones are somehow bad.

What many don't realize is that your hormones are your messengers. They allow your body to interface with every cell and vital system, as well as with the outside world. Hormones are your communication system, and you need clear communication within your body for it to run effectively. Without your sex hormones, you really don't have a foundation, for the rest of your hormones to be healthy.

Once you go through the change and you no longer have all your sex hormones available, you have other endocrine glands that will help out, even if you decide not to take hormone replacement therapy.

However, this isn't available if you're wearing all of those glands out too. Later in the book, we'll talk about how your other endocrine glands – the parts of your body that make hormones – are affected by the change.

Now let's talk about your sex hormones.

Estrogen is the fertilizer that feeds all of your tissues. She acts as a growth factor, and helps keep everything, including your body and your brain, juicy and vital. Did you know that memory and learning are both influenced by estrogen? Estrogen is the reason women are able to multitask, because it connects the two hemispheres of your brain.

By age one, female infants have better verbal skills and are better able to connect the left and right hemispheres of their brains than male infants. As you progress through childhood and then puberty, estrogen creates even greater connections between the right and the left half of your brain. Estrogen allows communication between the analytical aspect of your brain, and the part that's intuitive and artistic.

Estrogen also affects your moods, memory, and your ability to learn. It affects the linings of every body part: your mouth, your nose, your lungs, your gastrointestinal tract, your bladder, your vagina. For those linings to function normally, to be juicy and healthy, you need estrogen. The quality, health, thickness, and texture of your hair– that's all estrogen. Your nails also need estrogen. Because estrogen is one of your main growth factors, it prevents you from losing excessive bone.

Estrogen helps you make collagen so that all your tissues attach firmly onto your skeleton, and your skin, muscles, and bladder don't sag. Like I've said, estrogen is a fertilizer. But because it's a fertilizer, estrogen doesn't know the difference between the weeds and the roses. It'll fertilize everything, so if you have something cooking in your body, let's say breast cancer, estrogen will feed it.

Progesterone is the gardener, and it knows the difference between the roses and the weeds. Since estrogen is such a potent fertilizer, you make 10 to 50 times more progesterone than estrogen when you're reproductively viable and having periods.

You might have seen charts diagraming the menstrual cycle. If the measurements between the hormones were equal, progesterone would be off the chart, because you make that much more of it. Progesterone also acts as a growth factor, helping to grow myelin sheaths, the insulation around your nerves.

But the main function of progesterone is to control your DNA. Progesterone notices when you have cells that are outliving their welcome, like your uterine lining. When it's ready to shed because you're not pregnant, it's progesterone that triggers your period.

Progesterone turns on a gene called the "p53 gene," which is the cell death gene. It does this when it notices cells are no longer needed, for example your breasts, where cells develop every month in order to potentially produce breast milk if you are pregnant. But if you don't become pregnant during the menstrual cycle, progesterone turns all that growth off. You need to have enough progesterone to counterbalance your estrogen, plus you need extra progesterone because your adrenals use it to make cortisol.

Testosterone is the motivator, and is an androgen, or a male hormone. Estrogen helps bind or handcuff testosterone to prevent masculinization – like male pattern baldness and facial hair. Testosterone is anabolic, meaning it stimulates cell growth. It helps increase your strength, your bone density, and your muscle tone. In your brain, testosterone fuels your motivation.

All three sex hormones – estrogen, progesterone and testosterone – help keep you healthy.

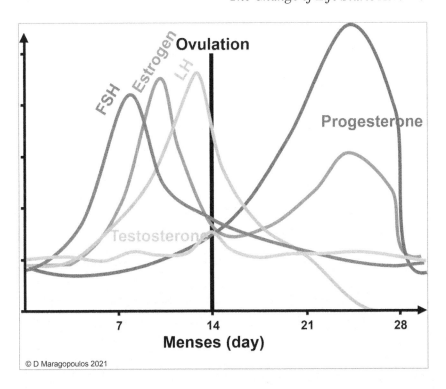

So how do you know if you have enough sex hormones?

Measuring hormones is not easy.

By the time my hormonally challenged patients consult with me, they've been out of balance for a long time. You can't function without any hormones, so it's unusual to find much from laboratory testing. And of course, no one comes to me with a lab report of their healthy baseline to compare with where they are currently.

Let's say you come to me at 45 years of age, complaining of peri-menopausal symptoms. I guarantee that your hormone levels are low for you, but it may not show on a blood test or even saliva or urine test. What did your levels look like when you were 25 and hormonally competent? We don't have a basis for comparison.

For instance, normal estrogen ranges are very, very wide. The range of estrogen for the average woman is 40 to 400 nanograms per deciliter, depending on where she is in her menstrual cycle. That's a huge range.

So if you were on average, a 300 to 400 kind of woman who dropped to 100, and we only measured your estrogen levels, the lab is going to report that your estrogen levels are normal. But if we measured your FSH, or your follicle stimulating hormone, which is the pituitary hormone that stimulates your ovaries to ripen follicles which produce estrogen, your FSH is going to be high.

It's your hypothalamus that perceives your estrogen levels and says, "Hey, we're not getting enough estrogen. It's only a third of what we're used to getting. We need more." Your hypothalamus will stimulate your pituitary gland to make more follicle stimulating hormone, or FSH.

So, it's your elevated FSH, *not your estrogen level*, that indicates you're in perimenopause. Same with progesterone. Progesterone doesn't have as wide a variable as estrogen, but it is very precise in terms of when you make it. Women make the majority of their progesterone at the end of their cycle in their luteal phase, so it matters where in your cycle we're measuring your progesterone levels.

Luteinizing hormone (LH) is the pituitary hormone that stimulates ovulation. And it's the corpus luteum – the little cave left when one follicle ovulates – that produces progesterone. When progesterone is high, like during pregnancy, your hypothalamus perceives it and doesn't stimulate your pituitary gland to make more LH.

Since hypothalamus hormones cannot be measured, I look at pituitary hormones – FSH and LH – rather than measuring estrogen and progesterone to determine whether your hormones are in balance. And I look at your symptoms, your menstrual cycle, what your patterns were and where you are now, to determine where you are in the change.

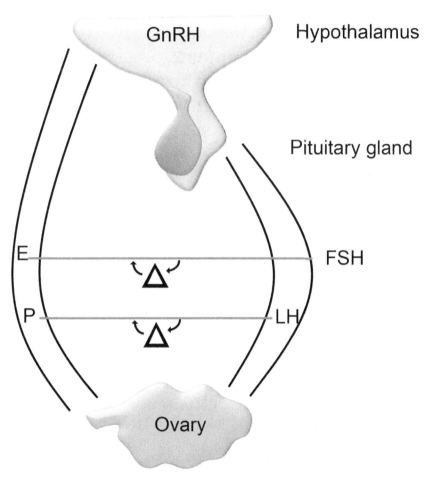

Identifying where you are in the change of life is the first step on your MAP....

Chapter 2

Where are You in the Change?

There are four main phases of the change of life: perimenopause, menopause, and postmenopause, plus premenopause. Yes, premenopause – the phase before perimenopause.

I'm going to talk about premenopause separately from perimenopause. Typically, the terms – premenopause and perimenopause – are interchangeable. But in the past 15 years, I've noted in my clinical practice this earliest phase, usually starting when women are in their 30s, when their hormones begin getting seriously out of balance.

These young women are really suffering because premenopause is not widely recognized. Let's talk about the symptoms of premenopause before we move into perimenopause, then menopause, and finally postmenopause. See if you can recognize where you are in the change.

Premenopause

Premenopause is usually between the ages of 35 and 40. I've seen women experience it a little bit earlier than 35. I haven't seen it in anybody older than 45.

If you're premenopausal, your main hormone issue is very low progesterone compared to estrogen, meaning you're estrogen dominant. Now, if we check your progesterone levels to see if you're fertile, you may have enough progesterone to conceive, indicating you're still ovulating, but you have a decreased progesterone to estrogen ratio. If we had checked you 10 or 15 years earlier, we would see that you have less progesterone now.

So what are you experiencing? You're bloated and you have breast pain. Your periods are all over the place.

If this is happening, you're not making enough progesterone to regulate your cycles, so your periods become unpredictable. When you do get your period, it tends to be really heavy with clotting. You may even spot before and after your period.

Let's say your typical period was five days of bleeding. Day one isn't so bad. Day two is the heaviest. On day three, it goes down. On days four and five, it kind of peters out. Now, you've got two or three days of spotting, before a super heavy flow for three to four days, followed by two to three days of spotting afterwards. You're wearing protection for seven to ten days out of the month.

Your periods may become more painful, because when you're estrogen dominant, you make a lot more prostaglandins which cause inflammation and painful uterine contractions. You may be passing clots. Your periods are heavy and uncomfortable. Your PMS symptoms are increased, or if you've never had PMS before, all of a sudden you do. Now, you're cranky. You're irritable. You cry at the drop of a hat. You never had any issues with your moods before, but now, they're all over the place.

You never had pre-bloating. You never had painful breasts before. You never had a change in your bowels, where you went from constipated to really loose stools and then you started bleeding. Now, you're experiencing all of these symptoms. Or maybe you had all those symptoms, but now they're worse. You never had premenstrual headaches, but now you have them. This is because you're estrogen dominant, and you don't have enough progesterone to counterbalance your estrogen.

Your fertility is decreasing as you're running out of eggs. We can measure this with a blood test by measuring anti-mullerian hormone (AMH). AMH actually measures your ovarian reserve, or how many eggs you have left. You're born with about a million eggs, and by the time puberty starts you have 300,000 eggs left. Every menstrual cycle, about 15 follicles mature under the influence of FSH – follicle stimulating hormone. But only one, or in very rare cases two, get to be the egg of the month and actually ovulate. And when your follicle numbers get low enough, your AMH will start to fall, meaning you just have a lot less oocytes (eggs) available.

Now, the egg of the month that ovulates to become the potential baby is not the issue. It's all those follicles that *could* be the egg of the month that should be producing estrogen that cause your symptoms. And when you do ovulate, your corpus luteum isn't producing enough progesterone, causing you to become estrogen dominant.

If you're under 40 years old and your FSH is in the menopausal range (over 30) and your AMH is low, indicating you've run out of eggs, it's called "premature ovarian failure." It's not called menopause at that point, but once you're over 40, we call it menopause. I believe in the next 5 to 10 years, we'll be moving the age of menopause down because we're starting to see premature ovarian failure in women in their late 20s to mid-30s.

Perimenopause

Perimenopause refers to the transitional time before your very last period. Perimenopause is also called the climacteric. During perimenopause, things are getting a little hectic because you're running out of hormones. Between 40 and 50 years old, your progesterone is low and your estrogen is beginning to decline. While you're still estrogen dominant because you have too much estrogen compared to progesterone, you also have symptoms of low estrogen.

Your moodiness has increased. You're experiencing brain fog. Your periods are unpredictable. They get super close together for a few months, going from maybe a 28-day cycle to 24, 22, 20 days, and then you skip a whole cycle. You may skip a whole month or two, and then have a really heavy period. This may happen two or three times a year.

Skipping periods is one of the classic signs of perimenopause. Polycystic ovary syndrome (PCOS) has similar period problems. If you have PCOS, you tend to be estrogen dominant and may not be ovulating regularly. This means that you will skip some periods, but unlike perimenopause, you have other markers that indicate PCOS. Your DHEA levels are high, your testosterone is high, and you have metabolic issues.

The biggest issue for my perimenopausal patients is they're having a hard time managing many aspects of their life, including stress, weight, relationships, and careers. Everything is more difficult for them, which has to do with their declining estrogen. Remember that estrogen connects the two halves of your brain. When you were younger, you were able to multitask and take care of so many things – your home, your job, your kids, your pets, your relatives, everything. And now, you can't. That's one of the signs of perimenopause – an inability to manage your normal daily stressors.

During perimenopause, you have all the symptoms of premenopause, but you also start to have classic menopausal symptoms because of lower estrogen levels. You may get hot flashes and night sweats. It may feel more like flushes where you feel hot and then chilled. You may not get the classic bright red flush and begin sweating on your chest and head, but you may just feel a little overheated.

You may notice that you're gaining weight. Now, typically the weight gain is going to be in the female distribution: your bust, your hips, your thighs, your butt, your curves. But you may also notice your waist is getting a little thicker, and that never really happened before. That's part of the perimenopausal hormone shift.

You're not going to sleep as deeply. You're going to have trouble falling asleep because you're making less progesterone, which means you're not making as much GABA (a calming neurotransmitter) so you can't settle down enough to fall asleep easily.

Because your estrogen is declining, you may wake up in the middle of the night feeling anxious. You may have to urinate, maybe not. You're just angsty, your thoughts are racing, and your heart might be racing too.

You might also start to notice that your brain is a little foggy. You walk into a room and you can't remember what you're looking for. You're having trouble dealing with your emotions. You're definitely moodier. For me, it was the moodiness that was the worst part of perimenopause. I didn't have the rest of the symptoms, but the moodiness was bad enough that my husband said something. I really needed to take the reins of my own change because it was affecting my relationships.

The one symptom that I have seen in perimenopause that totally gets overlooked is what I call the "hormonal flu." Honestly, I wasn't sure about this symptom until I experienced it myself. It feels like you're getting the flu. You feel feverish, achy, and super tired. It usually happens a day or two before your period, and then your period starts and you're fine. It's a very strange symptom. And I experienced the hormonal flu three times before I realized it was part of perimenopause. I could have sworn I was catching something. Even your glands can feel swollen.

This hormonal flu is the result of your declining progesterone and estrogen. You have a lot more inflammation, which becomes accentuated the closer you get to your period. The inflammatory reaction is your immune system creating an immune response, which makes you feel flu-like symptoms. It's not a common symptom, but it indicates that you're probably in perimenopause.

Your follicle stimulating hormone (FSH) is fluctuating because your estrogen is up and down. Some months, you make enough estrogen and your breasts are super sore and you're bloated and gain water weight, then you have a heavy period. Other months, you make less estrogen and you have lighter bleeding, or maybe even skip your period altogether.

So, trying to get an accurate FSH on a perimenopausal woman is hard. I recommend your FSH be measured on day three to five of your cycle (day one is the first day you bleed), because that's when your FSH should be at its lowest. If your FSH is elevated, it means your estrogen levels are starting to fall. So if we catch one elevation, that means you're perimenopausal, but because of your rollercoaster hormones, we could check it three or four times and still not catch it.

There are also gynecological issues that occur in perimenopause. If you have a tendency towards fibroids, they're growing now because of your estrogen dominance. Ovarian cysts are another normal occurrence during perimenopause.

Back in the early 90's, I worked in a women's health clinic where we did ultrasounds, and commonly found cysts in our 40-50 year old patients. More often than not, the surgeon would remove the cysts laparoscopically but they would keep coming back. I noticed that these were all perimenopausal women, so I started taking a wait-and-see approach. Most of the time, the cysts would resolve on their own. Years later, research showed that ovarian cysts were a normal part of going through the perimenopausal transition.

For the most part, these cysts can just be watched. They do not need to be surgically drained or removed. They're very common, and occur because your FSH is rising and overstimulating your ovarian follicles. The follicles get bigger than usual, and because you don't have enough progesterone to shut them down, you may have a follicle from the month before that continues to get overstimulated two or three months down the line, causing a cyst to form. If they're painful, or if they rupture or twist, they need to be dealt with surgically, but most of the time, ovarian cysts can be monitored through ultrasound. They usually resolve on their own.

Fibroids are different. Fibroids erupt from the structural tissue of the uterus. They can grow on the outside or inside of the uterus, or within the muscle layer of the uterus itself. They're benign tumors, but they can grow to be really big. They can grow so big that it looks like you're pregnant. It's not uncommon to see fibroids emerge in perimenopause due to estrogen dominance.

I have a fibroid that started growing in perimenopause. It's about the size of a golf ball. I'm very sensitive to my own body, so I felt this little fibroid pushing on my left sciatic nerve. Even when I had an ultrasound, the tech wasn't seeing it. So I told her, "You need to do a vaginal ultrasound. The abdominal ultrasound is not going to show it. I'll guide you and tell you where you need to go in order to see it." With my guidance, she was able to see it. But that's because I know my body really well. My fibroid erupted because even though my estrogen was declining, my progesterone was even lower. When estrogen is out of balance with progesterone, it feeds abnormal growth, like fibroids. Since menopause, my fibroid has shrunk without treatment.

Stress will induce an early change of life. If you are under a tremendous amount of stress in your 30s and into your 40s, you will go through perimenopause sooner than expected. Why? Stress robs your ovaries of progesterone to fuel adrenal production of the stress hormone, cortisol, and you will go through the change faster because your hypothalamus gets so worn out by constantly working to deal with your stressors.

I've seen many times, where in spite of their mothers' onset of menopause in their 50s, my patients have had such a tremendous amount of stress over a period of time, that they go through the change way earlier, sometimes up to 10 years earlier. It's not uncommon.

In my own patient population, the age of menopause is dropping. I believe it's because of the stress that women are under in our modern life. We are stressed by having to take care of so much. Even if our spouses, or partners want to be helpful, we tend to do most of the heavy lifting when it comes to taking care of the kids, the pets, the house, or our aging parents, all while working full time jobs.

By the time you're perimenopausal, you may have children at home, possibly moody teenagers. You may be taking care of your aging parents. You're part of the sandwich generation, where by having children later and with parents living longer, both generations are dependent on you. Plus, you have a job, and you still have to take care of the household. And your spouse may be going through his own change too – andropause. So, of course, you're being taxed physically, mentally, and emotionally, which makes going through menopause even more challenging.

Perimenopause taxes all women. Some of my most stressed patients are childless women who take on the burden of the rest of their family, sometimes handling way more than they should at work, because they don't have children. And if they're single, the burdens can be even heavier. Everyone in their life assumes they have the time and energy to be there for them, yet the support is one-sided.

This is just one of the many reasons why supporting yourself through the change is paramount, especially when so many others depend on you!

Menopause

Menopause literally means your "last period." You're menopausal if you haven't had a period for at least a year, or 13 menstrual cycles. Your FSH is over 30, and it stays over 30. Typically, menopause happens between the ages of 45 and 58.

Menopause is characterized by low progesterone, low estrogen, and declining testosterone. It's not bottomed out yet, but testosterone is declining.

Typically, insomnia is a huge issue in menopause. You're tired and irritable. Plus you're itchy, and you start having weird skin issues. You experience crazy itchiness that has no rash related to it, so you scratch until you have hives. You may be getting hot flashes now, as it's the most common symptom, and includes night sweats and chills. Your body temperature goes from super hot to super cold, so you find yourself ripping off your clothes, and then having to put a sweater on. You don't match the temperature of the room or what's comfortable for everyone else around you.

One of the things that I find most disconcerting now that I'm menopausal, is that my exam room is not very big. So when I'm consulting with a patient who needs the exam room a little warmer because she's getting undressed for a full exam, the room is too warm for me. So I'm always wearing layers of breathable materials like cotton or silk.

Now I finally understand what my mother was talking about when she complained about wearing polyester. She said her skin was suffocating. It was menopause. Sorry, Mom!

Sometimes during her consultation, my patient and I get so excited about finally discovering the root of her multiple health issues that we both get flushed and overheated!

Women having simultaneous hot flashes is not unusual. In my late 30's, I was the president of the California Coalition of Nurse Practitioners. Most of the nurse practitioners on this volunteer board were middle-aged women. Because of this, there was a lot of hot flashing going on. They would get really excited about something we were dealing with politically – to improve our practice or help our patients – and it was like a wave of hot flashes around the board table.

A shared pheromone response happens when you get excited about something, and if your hormones are a little bit out of balance, you're going to have a vasomotor response, which is the medical term for hot flashes. This is especially prone to happen if you're in a group of women going through the change too.

By menopause, it's getting harder to lose those extra pounds. If you haven't already seen some weight gain in perimenopause, you may start seeing some now. Most of the fat is deposited in your belly. You're getting thicker from your armpits down to your hips. Your breasts are getting bigger, and now you have back fat where your bra strap seems to be cutting into your flesh.

This is the result of your hormones being out of balance, creating a sluggish metabolism. You're in survival mode, and your hypothalamus is trying to save all those calories in a fat buoy around your middle because it perceives you're in danger.

Your brain is super foggy now. You're having trouble concentrating. You're having trouble focusing. It's difficult to start something new, learning-wise, because you don't retain new information as easily.

Your vagina is getting dry. You may notice that urine is leaking a little bit when you cough or sneeze, especially if you've had children. Even if you haven't birthed babies vaginally, you may experience some stress incontinence. This is because without enough estrogen, you don't have as much collagen to hold your bladder up.

Estrogen creates a lush vagina. When I do a wet mount on a patient, or gently scraping the lining of the vagina to examine the cells and any discharge for signs of infection, I can see the health of vaginal cells under the microscope. The vaginal cells of a healthy, young woman are plump little squares with a tiny nucleus in the middle. These squamous cells line everything – your skin, mouth, and vagina.

When women become menopausal, their vaginal cells start shriveling. They almost look like raisins, because without adequate estrogen, the cells lose fluid, which causes vaginal dryness. Vaginal infections are more common during this time because your vaginal flora, the beneficial bacteria, thrive in a healthy vagina. Healthy squamous cells hold a lot of glycogen, which is stored sugar that feeds protective lactobacillus acidophilus. So without adequate estrogen, you may develop vaginal dysbiosis, meaning an imbalance in your vaginal flora.

During menopause, you're a little more prone to yeast infections and bacterial vaginosis, which is an overgrowth of non-beneficial bacteria in the vagina. You may get more bladder infections because the collagen of your bladder neck is weaker. You may also notice that your libido is dipping. You just don't even feel like having sex anymore, and you're not lubricating as well. All of this is because your hormones are dropping.

You start noticing skin changes. You'll see dark spots, which is melanin that was damaged from sun exposure when you were younger. Now that you make less collagen and your skin is getting thinner, you can see the damage. You may also have light spots, or areas that look faded. This especially occurs on your legs, where you lose melanin because you don't have enough estrogen to stimulate normal melanin production.

You might notice skin tags, which could start early in perimenopause, due to estrogen dominance. These tags may be the same color as your skin or a little darker, and almost look like a mole but they're sticking out. They're not dangerous, but if they get irritated and bleed, you need to get them checked.

You may notice that you experience more depression or anxiety, especially if you already have a mood disorder. If you had postpartum depression, you're at a higher risk of having depression during menopause, because your brain doesn't tolerate the hormone changes as well.

The main sign of menopause is not having a period for at least a year. From here, you'll begin to experience the postmenopause phase.

Postmenopause

Postmenopause begins two years after your last period. You may be over 60 at this point, although if you start menopause in your late 40's, you may only be in your 50's when you reach the last phase of the change.

Postmenopause is characterized by having low everything: low progesterone, low estrogen, and low testosterone.

If you hadn't noticed wrinkles before, they're obvious now. You might even notice whiskers, especially on your chin. Your age is starting to show. You've lost enough collagen that you're seeing wrinkles because of low estrogen. The whiskers are prominent because even though your testosterone is low, your estrogen is lower, causing hair to grow in unwanted places.

You may also feel weakness, like you've lost the strength you used to have. Postmenopausal weakness is caused by low sex hormones, particularly testosterone. You're losing muscle tone, and you may have bone loss. While estrogen levels fall drastically in menopause and bone is lost rapidly, it's progesterone, testosterone, DHEA, and human growth hormone that help you grow bone.

Now that your progesterone and testosterone are low, and at this point, your adrenal hormones and growth hormone levels are lower, you're not laying down new bone as fast as you're losing it. You may develop osteoporosis, especially if you didn't take measures earlier to help slow down bone loss.

You may notice that you actually have some hair loss as well. If your hair is thinning in the male pattern, at your temples and crown, it's being caused by the testosterone dominance of menopause which initiates hair loss. Most postmenopausal women notice thinning all over – you have less hair follicles per centimeter. You're losing more hair because you don't have the growth factors, particularly estrogen, to grow those follicles. Your hair is stimulated by estrogen and thyroid hormone, particularly T_3. Without estrogen, you don't have enough T_3 to keep your hair nice and lush.

You may notice at this point that sex is not only painful because your vagina is dry, but you have trouble with orgasm. That's because all your sex hormones have dropped, and you have low progesterone, estrogen, and testosterone. Without adequate estrogen, you're not making as much oxytocin as you used to, and oxytocin is really the hormone of orgasm.

You may lose some vitality, meaning you just don't feel as strong and healthy as you used to. You're a little more vulnerable to infections. Cancers are starting to show up at this point, like skin cancers from past sun exposure. Other types of cancers may start to show up as well. It doesn't mean that all of a sudden you turn a certain age and a tumor grows. It means that because your hormones have fallen, your immune system isn't protecting you like it used to.

Even when you're younger, you have cancerous or precancerous cells developing all the time. But youth insures viable hormones to keep your immune system strong, so your immune cells are constantly going after those cancer cells that want to take over the kingdom. That's basically what cancer is – crazy, mutinous cells.

When you reach the postmenopausal period, you've lost sex hormones that help to support your immune system, so cancers start to grow. It's really important that you're getting all your screening tests done at this point, just to make sure that nothing is growing. It's also super important that you're taking lifestyle measures to help prevent cancer. Later in the book, we're going to discuss the lifestyle changes that need to be adopted to thrive in the postmenopause phase.

Postmenopause is when chronic illnesses begin to show up. Your blood pressure may be high, or your cholesterol is up. You may have developed insulin resistance or type 2 diabetes. You may have arthritis – the "wear and tear" kind, called osteoarthritis. Autoimmune disorders may or may not get worse during the postmenopausal period. Some autoimmune conditions get better, but some can actually get worse.

You may have pain in your muscles, joints, or bones that doesn't make sense to any of these other chronic illnesses. And, again, because your sex hormones are low, you have a lot more inflammatory cytokines. Cytokines are little tiny immune hormones, or cell messengers like interferon and interleukin that talk to each other.

Those cytokines, the inflammatory ones, cause inflammation in your joints, muscles, and bones for no reason at all. You may also have wear and tear issues that are now showing up. Perhaps you injured yourself while skiing a long time ago, and now that old knee injury is bothering you. Because you've run out of cartilage, your joint no longer makes the lubrication fluid that helps it function effectively, resulting in more pain.

You may also notice some neuropathy. Neuropathy means that you have strange pains and sensations, usually in your peripheral nerves. If you're diabetic or insulin resistant, you're more prone to neuropathy, and being postmenopausal makes it worse. Estrogen allows nerves to communicate faster, and progesterone builds the myelin sheath so that the nerves don't misfire. Now that you have low progesterone and low estrogen, your nerve communication is off.

Urinary tract infections are common in postmenopausal women. Because of the lack of collagen, your bladder starts sinking down on its neck, causing you to have a little bit of residual urine, even after you urinate. Bacteria can easily migrate up your short urethra to multiply in that little pool of urine and infect your bladder.

Between the ages of 65 and 75, women go through what I call a "second menopause" despite being postmenopausal. If their adrenal glands were doing a really good job of producing DHEA and pregnenolone, the mother hormones that convert into testosterone and estrogen, these adrenal hormones will carry them through menopause. Then, in your sixth decade when your adrenals naturally go through their own pause – adrenopause – you might experience symptoms of menopause again. The hot flashes, insomnia, and night sweats return. It feels like menopause all over again.

Women who are really healthy through their younger years may have some symptoms during menopause, but they do pretty well overall. They have healthy adrenals because they've been taking care of themselves. They eat well. They've been supporting their hypothalamus. They have good stress reduction techniques. They use prayer and meditation. They're connected to nature. They stay active. They have good sleep habits. Their adrenals last longer so they go through the change much more gracefully, but eventually their adrenals will decline too.

When my husband and I went back to our motherlands, Greece and Italy, we noticed, particularly in Italy, that the women tend to age very gracefully. It was very difficult to tell the difference between a 50-year-old and a 70-year-old in terms of her face, posture and the tone of her body. I think a lot of that has to do with how Italians handle stress.

Italians have a great family connection, and a great community connection. They're not as driven to get things done as we are here in the United States. They handle stress more gracefully so their adrenals last longer. They go through menopause at the same age as we do, but they have more sex hormone reserve. Their adrenals carry them with the hormones that they need to gracefully go through the change.

Women in this country are so stressed that their adrenals cannot possibly support them through menopause. Adrenal fatigue is not uncommon in 20 to 30-year-old women, and becomes more common in your 40s. If your adrenals are not functioning optimally when you go through perimenopause, menopause is going to be more drastic, and postmenopause is going to be complicated by chronic debilitating illnesses.

That's why women need a personalized Menopause Action Plan to be able to head these issues off at the pass.

ACTION ∼ Are you premenopausal, perimenopausal, menopausal or postmenopausal?

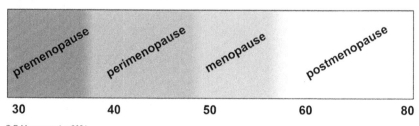

© D Maragopoulos 2021

Part Two

Learning the Lay of the Land

Chapter 3

What Happens in the Change?

Right before Dot celebrated her 40th birthday, she began waking up in the middle of the night sweaty, her heart racing, her thoughts anxious. Her doctor gave her benzodiazepines, but they didn't help. She was so irritable, and couldn't seem to handle stress like she used to. Her libido was lackluster. She put on 15 pounds. Then she started skipping periods. Her doctor said it was stress-related, and wanted to give her an antidepressant.

Dot's a smart, well-read woman, and insisted on bloodwork before taking another pill. Her doctor insisted she was too young for menopause and didn't want to order an FSH. Dot persisted, and sure enough, she was in full-blown menopause. That's when she came to me. Dot had all the classic symptoms of menopause, but she just didn't fit the age. Thankfully, she listened to her own intuition and got the help she needed. The first thing I did for Dot was educate her on how her body works, and what was happening since she'd entered menopause.

I believe education is the key to empowered menopause. I think education is the key to a lot of things, but definitely, to be empowered during the change of life, you need to be educated about what is happening, what's going to happen, and how you're going to deal with it. The more information that you gather about the change, the more prepared you'll be. Then you won't be shocked by any symptoms that might come up, nor by any changes in your body.

You'll know what's happening, and you'll know how to treat it . Now, if you're already through menopause, it's not too late to understand more about what's going on, and how you can treat your symptoms going forward. And most importantly, you can prevent chronic illnesses that are exacerbated by having your hormones bottom out in the change.

All of the symptoms that you suffer from in menopause are related to your declining sex hormones, and those declining sex hormones affect your hypothalamus. Your hypothalamus, a small gland in the center of your brain, is the master controller of all of your hormones.

The decline of your sex hormones causes your hypothalamus to get of balance, which is bad. That's because your hypothalamus controls so many vital systems of your body – your sleep, your temperature, your weight set point, your hunger and satiety, your metabolism, how fast you burn energy. Your hypothalamus controls your thyroid hormones, your adrenal hormones, your glucose metabolism, your digestion and detoxification. It also controls the function of your immune system, your memory, your concentration, your focus, and your moods.

Hypothalamic dysfunction causes the majority of symptoms in menopause.

After three decades of menstruating, your hypothalamus becomes reliant on your sex hormones – estrogen, progesterone and testosterone. Your sex hormones are the base of your pyramid of health. They need to be stable for your body to function optimally. When your sex hormones start bottoming out, it throws your hypothalamus off. All the symptoms you're experiencing occur due to the misfiring of the vital systems that your hypothalamus controls.

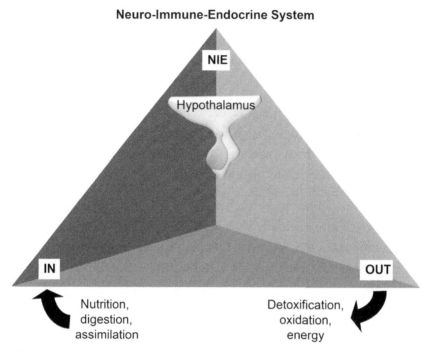

The majority of times, when you consult with a health care provider, they're just going after symptom control. Yet, if you focus on getting your hypothalamus calmed down and balanced, you won't be chasing symptoms.

Your hypothalamus can tolerate a slow decline in hormones, but it does not tolerate a rapid decline like menopause. When your hormones bottom out during the change, your hypothalamus becomes dysfunctional.

Your hypothalamus regulates your hormones through a sensitive feedback system. Your sex hormones are regulated by the hypothalamic-pituitary-ovarian axis. That's the communication between your hypothalamus, which is the master controller, the boss, the CEO, and your pituitary gland, which is middle management, and your ovaries, the workers. It's a negative feedback system, meaning that when estrogen is low, your hypothalamus stimulates your pituitary to produce more FSH. When progesterone is low, the hypothalamus stimulates your pituitary to produce more LH. It's a constant feedback mechanism, and when your hormones get out of balance, there's miscommunication.

Your hypothalamus is the link between your endocrine hormone system and your nervous system. It maintains all of your homeostasis, or your internal body balance, and it produces both releasing hormones as well as inhibiting hormones.

Your hypothalamus produces master hormones that get your endocrine glands to actually release their hormones. It also produces master hormones that stop the production of your hormones. Your hypothalamus is the wizard behind the curtain controlling everything.

How did you get so hormonally out of balance?

First, you start running out of eggs. Remember, you were born with over a million eggs. By the time you reach puberty, you have about 300,000, and then 15-20 follicles develop every menstrual cycle with hundreds of other prefollicles wasted. Most women have 13 cycles a year, and are reproductive for about 30 years. So, eventually you run out of eggs.

As you're running out of eggs, your hormone production decreases. The more unspent follicles you have, the more hormones you can make. In your youth, you have a huge ovarian reserve, meaning you have more ability to make sex hormones. Ten years before you even go through menopause, you have a lot less hormonal reserve because you have fewer follicles that might become the egg of the month and ovulate.

While estrogen is produced by the developing follicles, progesterone is only produced if you ovulate. Progesterone is produced by a transient endocrine gland called the *corpus luteum*. It's the little cave that's leftover after the egg pops out. Your ovaries make 95% of your body's progesterone needs in the luteal phase of your menstrual cycle – between ovulation and your period. Your adrenal glands produce only 5% of your progesterone.

Second, stress affects how hormonally challenged you are going to be through the change. Stress will rob your ovaries of progesterone. Your adrenal glands use progesterone to make cortisol, the stress hormone that fuels your fight-or-flight response. So, if you've been under a lot of stress, you've missed a lot of sleep, you've had major losses in your life, you've just experienced a major stressor, and especially if the stress has been happening over a long period of time, you're going to run out of sex hormones faster.

Stress causes you to go through the change sooner. Women are under more stress now than in previous generations, so we become hormonally challenged a lot younger.

Your adrenal glands sit right on top of your kidneys. When your adrenals produce cortisol, they also produce dehydroepiandrosterone (DHEA). Cortisol helps you metabolize glucose by releasing stored sugar called glycogen out of your liver and your muscles so that you can use it to fuel the fight-or-flight stress response.

Afterwards, you produce DHEA in order to metabolize protein and fat to heal you from the damage caused by the fight-or-flight. DHEA is a really important anabolic hormone, or a building hormone, to counterbalance the effects of cortisol. DHEA can be converted into testosterone and then into estrogen. That's why in countries that are not so stressed out, women tend to have a much more graceful menopause than women who live in more stressed countries. These women have more adrenal reserve with more DHEA, which means they have more estrogen on board longer.

The third factor that affects how you experience the change. How did you live your life? If you were exposed to lots of toxins, like xenoestrogens which are chemicals that take up receptor sites and compete with your natural estrogen, you're going to have less estrogen reserve, and you're going to have more issues.

What you've been eating can be an issue. If you've been nutritionally deficient for many years, you're not going to have the reserve you need to create enough sex hormones to stay healthy.

How active has your lifestyle been? Women who are more sedentary and do not have some kind of exercise program are not as hormonally balanced as active women are.

In our modern world, we're not as physically active as we used to be. You can buy a loaf of bread rather than baking it yourself. If you've ever kneaded raw dough, it takes a lot of upper body strength. With less physical activity in our daily existence, we need to exercise in order to stimulate our muscles and our metabolism. And exercise helps us metabolize our hormones better.

If you've missed sleep, it'll affect your hormones. Perhaps you don't go to bed on time. You're on a digital device after dusk, so you're being exposed to that blue screen, which is suppressing your ability to make melatonin. You don't have all the lights off in your bedroom. Maybe light is coming from the TV screen or a street light outside the window. Light also suppresses your melatonin production.

Perhaps you don't get deep sleep for at least seven to nine hours a night. Over time, that is going to affect your sex hormones. Sleep deprivation will definitely cause hypothalamic dysregulation, which will put you into a hormonally challenged state long before the change.

The fourth factor that affects your menopause experience is your mindset. Studies show that women who have a positive mindset towards menopause do better in menopause. It doesn't mean they don't have any symptoms. It just means their symptoms are a lot lighter, and they handle them better.

If you're constantly thinking, "Oh, my goodness, this horrible thing is happening to me. I'm going through the change. I'm going to get wrinkly and old and weak," you're more likely to manifest that which you believe.

But if you have a positive mindset where you say, "You know what? This is an empowering time for me. I'm done with this chapter of my life, and I'm moving onto the next. I really want to do life a little bit differently. I want to do something different that I have always wanted to do, and I can do that now," you're going to have a lot less symptoms. You're going to age more gracefully. You're going to see the good and not focus on the bad. Your mindset makes a huge difference in your experience of menopause.

The final factor influencing the hormonal imbalance of the change is how well your hypothalamus is functioning. Supporting your hypothalamus through the change is key. If you're able to support your hypothalamus early, starting in premenopause, you're probably going to delay menopause and you're going to handle stress better.

My personal experience has been by supporting my hypothalamus from the age of 38, I was able to put off menopause until 58. My three younger sisters who did not support their hypothalamus became menopausal by their mid forties, even though we have very similar lifestyles. We are like four peas in a pod, and are genetically similar. We've all eaten a Mediterranean diet, and we're all very active. Yet I supported my hypothalamus and went through menopause about the same age as our mother. I believe supporting my hypothalamus helped ease the toll stress took on my hormones and kept my body hormonally competent longer.

How do you know that you're going through the change?

Your FSH, or your follicle-stimulating hormone, is the classic measuring tool. It's a blood test that can show if you're menopausal. If your FSH is over 30, then you are menopausal. If you're still menstruating, andon day three to five of your menstrual cycle your FSH is over 15, you're perimenopausal.

But measuring FSH in a perimenopausal woman is kind of a crapshoot. Your FSH goes up and down according to what's going on with your estrogen. So, some months it's a little bit better, and other months it can be a little bit worse. As a clinician, I look at my patients' symptoms, and use the FSH as a baseline to see how much time they might have left to get hormonally balanced before going through menopause.

Later in the book, we're going to talk about how to treat all of these symptoms. For now, it's really important that you understand what's happening in your body first, so you know how to treat them.

ACTION ~ How high is your FSH?

Chapter 4

The Most Common Symptoms

Let's start with the six most common symptoms of menopause. Although there are over 40 symptoms associated with the change, I'm starting here because most women have either one or more of these symptoms. They can start as early as the premenopausal period, and definitely in perimenopause. Most women experience them in menopause, and these symptoms can extend through the postmenopause phase.

Hot Flashes

The number one symptom women have are hot flashes. Hot flashes, flushing, and night sweats are called vasomotor symptoms, because they involve the contraction and dilation of your blood vessels. Vasomotor symptoms are the most common, and. it has been estimated that 75-85% of postmenopausal women continue to have hot flashes.

Hot flashes are a very sudden feeling of heat, and can be accompanied by redness (flushing). The heat usually starts around your face and neck, and then spreads throughout your body. Hot flashes can be accompanied by sweating and a rapid heart rate, or tachycardia. So, your heart's racing. You're sweating. Your cheeks and chest are bright red. You're overly hot compared to the temperature of your environment. It could be freezing cold, and you can still be having hot flashes.

Vasomotor symptoms tend to last for about one to two years after menopause, and rarely last for more than 10 years. Your core body temperature is best measured rectally or orally, not underneath your arm, and not by checking your ears or the skin on your forehead. Your internal thermostat is controlled by the front part of your hypothalamus called the anterior hypothalamus.

Your anterior hypothalamus is home to the master hormone, gonadotropin releasing hormone or GnRH. So, the hormone that controls estrogen and progesterone is in the same place that your body temperature is controlled. It's no wonder when your estrogen levels fall, your core body temperature gets a little bit off. It's right in the same nuclei.

If my hypothalamus needs to raise my body temperature because it's cold outside, I'm going to have an increase in metabolism. I'm also going to experience peripheral vasoconstriction, where my blood vessels get really tight. That way, my blood stays in my core, feeding my vital organs.

If my hypothalamus needs to lower my body temperature, because I'm running and overly heated, my blood vessels experience vasodilation, meaning the blood vessels get wider, and there's a flushing into my skin, and I start sweating. That's normal. That's not hot flashes.

With hot flashes, you have both an increased metabolism, like a raise in body temperature, and you have vasodilatation and sweating. It's very much a dysfunction of the hypothalamus' ability to regulate your body temperature.

In menopausal women, our upper threshold of temperature is lowered, meaning we can't take super high temperatures. Everyone around me always wants to turn on heaters, and I prefer to have the rooms a little bit cooler. One thing I do is wear breathable clothing. Cotton and silk, rather than synthetic fibers, makes a big difference in keeping body temperature a little more stable.

A lower temperature threshold in menopause is because estrogen is depleted, yet hot flashes can start in perimenopause. During this time, you're not ovulating regularly, so luteinizing hormone is not surging and you can start having hot flashes. So, it's not just estrogen depletion that causes hot flashes. It's the lack of LH surges.

Remember that hypothalamic GNRH controls luteinizing hormone surges, as well as follicle stimulating hormone, which stimulates estrogen. The depletion of your sex hormones and the shift in the hypothalamic master control hormones affect your body temperature.

Insomnia

Insomnia is the second most common symptom of the change. Sometimes, insomnia is caused by night sweats and nocturnal hot flashes. In addition, if your body temperature threshold is lowered, and when you're running hot, it's very hard to make melatonin. You need a lower body temperature at night in order to make enough melatonin to sleep soundly.

So, it's hard to stay asleep. The most common insomnia symptom for menopausal and postmenopausal women is not trouble *falling* asleep, it's *staying* asleep. You tend to wake up between 1:00 and 4:00 AM, depending on whether it's winter or summer. Sometimes you have to urinate, and sometimes you don't. But you have trouble falling back to sleep.

This is because you're experiencing a dip in your melatonin production. The range of sleep disorders during the change is pretty wide.

Before hormones are clinically low, 16-42% of premenopausal women suffer from some sleep disorders. Even if you're making reproductively active hormones, you can still have some sleep issues. And your ability to fall asleep and stay asleep is definitely going to change during your menstrual cycles.

As your hormones decline, your sleep issues will get worse. By perimenopause, 39-47% of women have insomnia. And by the time women become postmenopausal, up to 65% will have issues with falling and staying asleep.

We know ovarian hormones affect sleep disorders, so let's start by exploring progesterone's role in affecting sleep, seeing that it's the first hormone to bottom out when you become perimenopausal. Progesterone has a sedative effect, meaning it can make you sleepy and relaxed. It also has an anti-anxiety effect, meaning it can calm you down. Progesterone stimulates the production of non-REM-associated GABA. GABA is a neuropeptide that calms down your overly excited nervous system. Progesterone also stimulates GABA receptors – the doorways into your neurons – to allow GABA to get in. Progesterone acts very much like a benzodiazepine, like Xanax or Valium, to calm you down.

Progesterone can be a respiratory stimulant, so unlike a benzodiazepine or a sedative that will calm you down so much that you may not breathe well, progesterone not only calms you down, but it helps to actually stimulate your respirations. In fact, progesterone is used to treat sleep apnea.

Sleep apnea means you stop breathing for a tiny period of time while you're sleeping, which can be seen in a sleep study. Sleep apnea is more common if you're overweight, and becomes more common as you get older.

The other hormone that affects sleep disorders is estrogen. Now, estrogen is associated with the metabolism of many neurotransmitters

– norepinephrine, serotonin, acetylcholine – which affect your sleep patterns, particularly REM sleep. During the night, estrogen keeps your body temperature low so you can make enough melatonin to go into deep REM sleep.

It's not just estrogen and progesterone affecting your sleep. There's a natural decline of melatonin which affects women in the post-menopausal phase. Melatonin is pretty stable when you're premenopausal, perimenopausal, or even early menopausal. But by the time you're in your 60's and postmenopausal, you definitely have lower melatonin production.

If you have a mood disorder, anxiety, or depression, you're more likely to have sleep disorders when you're postmenopausal. Mood disorders affect your ability to produce an adequate amount of neurotransmitters, and those neurotransmitters affect your day/night cycles, leading to insomnia. And of course, all is made worse by your declining sex hormones.

Weight Gain

Weight gain is very common during the change of life. In the United States, the prevalence of obesity in 40 - 59 year old women reaches up to 65%. Over the age of 60, the prevalence rises to almost 74%. So, why do you gain weight through the change?

Biologically, weight gain can be a survival mechanism. If you have a little extra weight when you hit menopause, you're less likely to have as many symptoms, because you store estrogen in your fat cells. If you come into menopause underweight, you're going to be more symptomatic. So five percent above your ideal weight can actually be a good thing in terms of symptoms.

The reason that you gain weight during menopause is because of your declining hormones' effect on your hypothalamus. Your hormones affect your metabolism and your hunger. In particular, estrogen affects fat metabolism. It helps you lay down brown fat and burn white fat.

You didn't know that your body fat comes in colors? White fat is the fat we don't want. It's the fat around your belly. It's the fat that's impregnating your visceral organs and culminating on your liver, causing fatty liver. Brown fat, however, is the fat that gives you feminine curves.

Both male and female infants have brown fat around their neck, shoulders, and core to keep them warm. Through childhood, we burn up our brown fat. Then at puberty, under the influence of estrogen, girls lay down more healthy brown fat, particularly in their hips and thighs. But as we get older and more metabolically sluggish, we lay down more inflammatory white fat – mostly in our bellies.

Estrogen also affects your hunger and your satiety, because it directly acts on your hypothalamus neurons. These neurons make a large pre-hormone called proopiomelanocortin (POMC). Hypothalamic POMC controls your metabolism, including your hunger and satiety, your day/night cycle, your stress response, and your level of happiness. POMC also regulates your cellular activity.

Active cells burn more energy. By keeping hypothalamic POMC levels up, estrogen helps keep your cells active and helps burn energy stored in your white fat. Estrogen also affects how effective your thyroid hormones are within your cells. This is because POMC helps control thyroid hormone production. When you're going through the change, your hypothalamus reacts and asks, "What the heck is going on down there? Why aren't the ovaries producing estrogen?" It then responds accordingly by slowing down your metabolism. That way, you can store body fat to use for energy if you no longer can fend for yourself.

So you can thank your hypothalamus for the protection and survival mechanism in the form of midlife body fat. The only problem is that in our modern times, you probably will not suffer from hunger and need to burn that extra energy.

It's important to maintain your ideal body weight, and more so, your lean body mass – your muscles and bones – to make sure your hormones stay as stable as possible as you're going through the change. While you might need bioidentical hormone replacement therapy, supporting your hypothalamus will keep your hormones in balance longer, so your weight will not be such an issue when you're going through menopause.

Mood Swings

The next most common symptom of menopause are mood swings. Your hypothalamus controls your state of happiness, including the neurotransmitters that affect your level of anxiety. When your sex hormones decline, they affect your hypothalamus' ability to regulate serotonin, dopamine, acetylcholine, and norepinephrine – all the neurotransmitters that affect your moods.

When your estrogen and progesterone are bottoming out, you may experience increased levels of depression. You may feel sad and have less motivation. You just don't feel like doing anything. You feel kind of hopeless. You may cry more easily. You may also feel more anxious or worried all the time, notice your heart racing, and feel kind of panicked,, all because your hormones are lower.

Remember, progesterone acts as an anti-anxiety hormone. When it bottoms out, you're going to be more anxious. That's why peri-menopausal women often first notice a shift in their moods.

As a menopausal woman who has been taking bioidentical hormone replacement therapy, estrogen feels like the joy hormone to me. And for me, progesterone is definitely the calming hormone. Without progesterone on board, it's hard to stay calm.

However, without estrogen on board, it's hard to find joy in things. Estrogen also helps stimulate the neurotransmitters of creativity, so it's hard to feel motivated and creative when your estrogen levels are lower. Supporting your hypothalamus throughout the change can help you stay in balance to keep your moods stable.

If you have a history of mood disorders, you're going to have more mood swings going through the change, starting in perimenopause. This is why it's important to plan ahead and create your own MAP – your Menopause Action Plan.

Low Libido

The next most common symptom is low libido or low sex drive. However, it's important to remember that women's sexuality is influenced by more than hormones. Our sexuality is influenced by our mood, our energy, and our sense of well-being. And likewise, our hormones affect our sense of well-being, our energy, and our moods. It's not just estrogen or testosterone that's affecting our libido. It's also prolactin, oxytocin, and beta-endorphins, which are produced by your hypothalamus.

When your estrogen level is lower, you definitely don't have much of a sex drive. Estrogen affects your sexual arousal, how lubricated your vagina is, how good your partner smells to you, and how sensitive your skin, and particularly your erogenous zones, are to stimulation. Testosterone affects your drive, but it affects it more in terms of the ability to orgasm. So, if you don't have enough testosterone on board, it can sometimes be a little harder to orgasm.

Prolactin also affects your drive. Prolactin is the hormone that induces breast milk production in nursing mothers. It's also an important nocturnal hormone that helps control your immune function. If your prolactin levels are too high, you will have a super diminished sex drive, which makes sense biologically, because breastfeeding women have very high prolactin levels. Prolactin diminishes a nursing mother's sex drive and can help prevent ovulation, so that she doesn't conceive too early and tax the resources that should be going to her breastfeeding infant.

As women go into menopause, and especially postmenopause, they naturally have a rise in prolactin. Not high enough to make breast milk, but they produce enough prolactin that it blocks their sex hormone receptor sites. So whatever little estrogen and testosterone they may be making from their adrenal glands, they're not feeling it. They aren't getting that stimulus to have a sex drive in the first place.

Oxytocin is your cuddle hormone. It's the hormone that bonds you to your infant, your partner, and your loved ones. Oxytocin is released when you orgasm. It's oxytocin that gives you the big bang. However, it's oxytocin that you feel when you're hugging or kissing your partner, holding a baby, hugging a friend, or cuddling your pets. If it's a long enough hug, you're going to feel that good oxytocin vibe.

Oxytocin's role is to help us bond with others. And if your oxytocin becomes depleted like when you're going through menopause, you're not feeling particularly cuddly, nor do you regularly experience the big bang of orgasm.

Beta-endorphins are your happy neuro-hormones. I think of beta-endorphins like a big, yellow happy face. They just make everything feel better. My experience with beta-endorphins was as an athlete. If you exercise long enough, you get into this place I like to call *the zone*, where your hypothalamus is producing beta-endorphins at such a high level that you feel no pain, and everything feels amazing.

You can feel the effects of beta-endorphins when you're doing something that should be painful, like riding your bicycle for 100 miles, but you're not feeling it. It can cause a little bit of a high, so much so that you seek the feeling again and again, which is why certain activities, even athletic activities, can be a little addictive.

While your hypothalamus directs the production of prolactin and oxytocin, beta-endorphins are actually a byproduct of proopiomelanocortin (POMC). Recall how POMC is adversely affected by your low estrogen levels. Can you see how it's all connected?

You're menopausal. Your estrogen levels are falling. Testosterone's falling. Prolactin is rising. You're not making as much oxytocin, or as much beta-endorphins. So, of course, you're not thinking about sex. You're not as sexually arousable. You're having trouble reaching orgasm. Thankfully, your libido can be revived.

Brain Fog

Brain fog can start in perimenopause and gets worse throughout the change. You walk into the room, and you don't remember why you're there. You put something down, and you lose it. You can't remember names or certain words. Word loss is super common, and that's because estrogen stimulates a speedy neuron transmission, meaning nerves talk faster under the influence of estrogen.

With youthful levels of estrogen on board, you're rapidly crossing over the median of the brain, or the corpus callosum. You have a speedy connection between the left analytical brain and the right creative brain. You're able to multitask. As your estrogen levels fall, your brain becomes foggy, your memory diminishes, and it's harder to focus.

Brain imaging studies in 40 to 60 year old women from perimenopause through postmenopause exhibit the kind of changes that we would see in Alzheimer's patients. Does that mean menopause causes Alzheimer's? No. However, it does mean that the lack of estrogen causes the same changes that we see in people with Alzheimer's.

What we're seeing is a decrease in metabolic activity in the brain, and a higher deposition of amyloids, which are basically scar tissue in the brain, compared to premenopausal women. Estrogen is so important for your brain that when you lose it, the structure of your brain and its function changes. Thankfully, there are ways to keep your brain healthy through the change.

ACTION ~ Which symptom is most bothersome for you?

Chapter 5

Lesser Known Symptoms

In the midst of the pandemic, Tracy consults with me on Zoom. At 55, she's been on bioidentical hormone replacement therapy for a few years, but can't seem to get her dosing right, so sleeping through the night is near impossible. Her mother and older sisters had the typical hot flashes and night sweats that kept them from sleeping. She hasn't had hot flashes, so she's not even sure why her doctor started her on hormones.

She wonders about some other strange symptoms – could they possibly be related to menopause? Severe constipation, chronic dermatitis, nail fungus, joint pain. Laxatives haven't helped her constipation. None of the ointments her dermatologist has prescribed has cleared her skin. And cortisone shots did nothing for her joint pain.

I explain to Tracy how her declining sex hormones affect her hypothalamus, and how her hypothalamus controls her gut function, immunity, and inflammation. So yes, these strange symptoms are part of going through the change. Getting Tracy's hormones back in balance and her hypothalamus functioning optimally will help ease her constipation, heal her dermatitis, and relieve her joint inflammation. A better functioning immune system will help her finally clear the nail fungus. But first we need to get her sleeping through the night, which requires a reset of her hypothalamus.

Doesn't it seem like your body starts falling apart by the time you're 50? Your cholesterol rises, perhaps even your blood pressure. Your joints hurt. You get injured more easily. You can't seem to fight off infections, and old issues, like childhood eczema, crop back up.

The foundation of your health rests upon a functioning hypothalamus. Your hypothalamus has been reliant on reproductive levels of sex steroids for decades. Going through the change pulls the rug out from under your hypothalamus, leading to symptoms seemingly unrelated to menopause.

Most women know that insomnia and hot flashes are common in menopause. They suspect that their weight gain may be related to menopause. They know that their sex drive may be lowered due to menopause. And their mood swings have always been affected by their hormones.

There are less well known symptoms that are actually quite common for women going through the change, yet not well known enough by women or their healthcare providers.

Maybe you go to your doctor like Tracy did, and none of your odd symptoms are attributed to the fact that you're going through menopause. Instead, your doctor chases other potential etiologies or causes of these symptoms. Yet all of the symptoms of menopause are because your hormones are depleted and your hypothalamus is out of balance.

To help make sense of these oddball symptoms, I've organized them by which body system is affected. You'll see why it's so important to support your hypothalamus, because the majority of the symptoms are in that area.

When you reach menopause, your ovaries are finally retired. In medicine, we call it ovarian failure. You know you're going to run out of eggs eventually, so it's like retirement. You're no longer producing sex hormones.

All the hormonal changes of menopause affect almost all aspects of your health, so you can experience signs and symptoms in nearly every body system. There are estrogen and progesterone receptors throughout your body. Every body system has these receptors, and the lack of these sex hormones is affecting all of your body systems.

One of the reasons for writing this book is to educate you. After reading this book, and particularly if you choose to join our MAP workshop, you will have an honorary degree in managing your menopause. Understanding why you're experiencing these symptoms will help you deal with them more effectively.

Are you ready? Ok! Let's go over all the symptoms of the change, grouped by your body systems.

There are four categories of symptoms: hypothalamic, gastrointestinal, dermatological and connective tissue, and neurological.

Hypothalamic Responses to the Change

The six most common symptoms are all hypothalamic responses to the change: hot flashes/night sweats, low libido, weight gain, mood swings, brain fog, and insomnia. And there's so much more.

Restless leg syndrome can aggravate menopausal insomnia. If you had restless leg syndrome when you were pregnant, you have a 60% chance of experiencing restless leg syndrome in menopause.

There's definitely a correlation with the fluctuating hormones in pregnancy and the fluctuating hormones in menopause. While pregnancy is a high hormone state and menopause is a low hormone state, both cause a dysregulation in your hypothalamus and nervous system.

Restless leg syndrome is related to the estrogen dominance of pregnancy, as well as the estrogen dominance of perimenopause. By postmenopause, 69% of women perceive that their restless leg syndrome is worse than what it was before menopause. Restless leg syndrome can keep you awake at night, as it creates the urge to get up and move your legs.

Panic attacks are relatively common in postmenopausal women, and seem to be associated with stressful life events. We're all under stress, but life gets a little more stressful when you reach middle age, because you're dealing with elderly parents, as well as your career and perhaps adult children or grandchildren.

Postmenopausal panic attacks are also more common if you have medical comorbidities. Meaning if you're obese, you have diabetes, metabolic syndrome, heart disease, or any kind of autoimmunity, you're more likely to have issues with panic attacks. If you have had functional psychiatric impairment in any way, like mood disorders, menopause will affect your anxiety level, and may increase panic attacks.

Irregular periods are a hypothalamic response to the change. Remember that your hypothalamus produces GNRH, which controls ovarian function via a negative feedback system. Your hypothalamus-pituitary-ovarian axis becomes dysfunctional, which leads to menstrual irregularity. During perimenopause, your periods get closer and closer together, then start spacing out until you skip cycles.

Fatigue is definitely a hypothalamic response, because the hypothalamus controls your metabolism, or your cells' ability to create energy.

Autoimmune disorders can shift during the change. Your immune system is controlled by your hypothalamus, and estrogen boosts your immune system, so some autoimmune conditions get worse, while others get better in menopause.

For instance, lupus gets better in menopause. Reproductive women who have lots of estrogen on board tend to have more lupus symptoms. On the other hand, rheumatoid arthritis tends to get worse in early menopause, and definitely worse in postmenopause.

Allergies can get worse. Even if you've never had allergies before, you can start developing allergies during menopause. They may manifest in the skin, sinuses, or lungs. The odds of getting asthma are twice as high in women going through menopause.

Going through the change makes your immune system hyper-reactive. A hypersensitive immune system reacts to environmental agents like pollens, danders, foods, and even beauty products.

Because you're lacking estrogen, going through the change can increase your vulnerability to infections. Let's look at shingles for instance. Middle-aged women are the population most likely to develop shingles. Shingles is related to the varicella virus, which is the same virus that causes chickenpox. If you've been exposed to a child with chickenpox, or even a child who has been recently given the varicella vaccine, you are likely to develop shingles.

Why? Because as your estrogen level lowers, your body forgets to make enough antibodies against diseases that you already had or were vaccinated against. Even if you had chickenpox as a kid, now you make less antibodies, so you're not fighting off this virus when you get exposed to it by your grandchild. And as a result, you develop shingles.

When you're menopausal, your immunity is more cell-mediated than antibody dependent. Cell-mediated immunity is when your WBCs, also known as macrophages, engulf foreign invaders.

This is also why you have more hypersensitivity, allergies, and rashes. Your immune system is going after things in an aggressive manner, instead of making enough antibodies to tell your WBCs, "Hey, this is something we should be going after, but that's our own tissue, which we should leave alone."

Antibodies are a much more refined immune response than cell-mediated immunity. Yet, by the postmenopause phase, women have high cell-mediated immunity and low antibody response. If you give a postmenopausal woman estrogen, it'll improve her immune response and she'll make more antibodies. You can see how estrogen affects your immune system, and the lack of estrogen increases your risk of autoimmunity, as well as allergies, vulnerability to infections, and even cancer.

Gastrointestinal Responses to the Change

The change affects your digestive tract. Lots of menopausal women will complain, "I'm not digesting foods properly. I'm more sensitive to certain foods. I'm having indigestion, nausea, constipation, gas, bloating, or I have diarrhea after I eat."

Since your hypothalamus controls your hunger and satiety, and has neuroendocrine control of your gut motility, you're going to have gastrointestinal issues when it becomes dysregulated by your low hormone levels.

Most of the time, your healthcare provider will not relate your gut symptoms to menopause. You'll be worked-up for gastro-esophageal reflux disorder (GERD). Maybe you actually have gastroesophageal reflux disease, but your inflamed stomach and esophagus, even your inflamed sinuses and that annoying cough caused by silent GERD, are a result of your declining hormones.

Your sex hormones have receptor sites in all different cell types in the gastrointestinal system. They're in your liver, your pancreas, and your gastrointestinal tract from your stomach and small intestine, all the way to your colon.

Your gut contains estrogen, progesterone, and testosterone receptors. These sex hormones modulate the activities of the cells in your digestive tract, and influence their physiological processes.

This means that hormones influence how your liver functions, whether you make enough bile, and if it's dumped properly by the gallbladder. Hormones influence whether you make enough pancreatic enzymes, and whether you make enough stomach acid. Hormones influence peristalsis, which is the movement of your gastrointestinal tract.

Estrogen stimulates intestinal enzyme levels, and facilitates absorption, so that you can absorb nutrients from food. Progesterone inhibits the circular muscles as well as the longitudinal smooth muscles in the intestinal tract. It can cause your gut to slow down somewhat giving you time to fully digest and absorb nutrients.

Estrogen and progesterone can help to protect and heal your gastric lining. So if you're missing estrogen and progesterone, you don't have the enzymes to protect yourself against your own hydrochloric acid. It's not that you're making too much acid, it's just that you aren't protected properly from it.

Most menopausal women are hypochloric. Your stomach makes too little hydrochloric acid, so you don't digest proteins and fats properly. Because you don't have enough estrogen and progesterone to actually boost the mucosa cells in your stomach to make hydrochloric acid, and also to make enough mucus to protect you from your own acid, you end up developing gastritis and GERD.

Menopausal women also tend to have indigestion due to sluggish gallbladders. You don't dump enough bile to neutralize the acidic food passing from your stomach into your small intestine. Pancreatic enzymes need a neutral pH to digest protein, fat, and carbohydrates.

So your food just sits there fermenting, causing belching and bloating.

Since estrogen keeps the linings of your organs nice and juicy, when your levels drop in menopause, your bile ducts get dry and stick together. This is why gallbladder issues like gallstones and inflammation called cholecystitis are common during the change.

We also know that your hormonal status affects your gut flora. Your microbiome are the friendly bacteria in your gut that help you safely metabolize your hormones. Your gut flora is enriched with genes that synthesize steroid hormones, which includes your sex hormones. Synthesizing hormones is how they're broken down, so you can get rid of them through your bowel movements.

If you don't synthesize your hormones properly, you will recycle them, meaning your gut will reabsorb them into the bloodstream, which isn't good. In premenopause, not synthesizing your hormones properly will create an estrogen dominant state. In menopause, you're recycling the most toxic forms of your hormones, which increases your risk of inflammatory diseases and hormone-fed cancers.

Healthy microflora is critical to healthy hormone metabolism. Yet without adequate sex hormones, your microflora is not going to be as robust and diverse to keep you healthy. Estrogen helps make the cells of the intestines very rich and thick to provide homes for your beneficial bacteria. The microbiota, or gut flora, of postmenopausal women looks very similar to men, not healthy like in premenopausal women. However, if a premenopausal woman is obese, she's more likely to have unhealthy gut flora.

From perimenopause through postmenopause, women have a high prevalence of altered bowel function, including gastrointestinal complaints such as diarrhea, cramping, bloating, gas, acid reflux, gastritis, abdominal pain, and constipation.

Dermatological and Connective Tissue Responses to the Change

Let's move on to your skin, muscle, bones, and joints. Your skin includes your hair and nails, plus all the mucous membranes lining your mouth, nose, lungs, and gut. All of the structure and surfaces of your body, inside and out, are affected by the change.

Your skin is the largest non-reproductive target in which estrogens and androgens act. Dermatosis, a medical term for skin rashes and abnormal changes, is incredibly common in menopause. That's because estrogen is vital for healthy skin, and essential for skin hydration. Estrogen drives your skin to make glycosaminoglycans, which are long sugar protein molecules that create a protective barrier and hold fluid in.

Without estrogen, you don't have the increased oil production you need to keep your skin moist, nor are your skin cells able to retain adequate water. Estrogen also improves the barrier function of the top layer of the skin, called the stratum corneum, so that you don't get cut so easily or get infections so easily. As people get older, their skin gets thinner, and tearing and bruising happens more easily, because they don't have this protective barrier.

Hormones affect your hair. Abnormal hair growth and hair loss are common during the change. Hirsutism, or male-like body and facial hair, is also related to low estrogen. You need enough estrogen to bind testosterone, and when your levels fall in menopause, you may see whiskers on your chin and upper lip. Alopecia means you're losing your hair either in a male pattern baldness or generalized thinning.

The issue with hair loss comes from both low estrogen and androgen dominance. Testosterone inhibits hair follicle growth, which can cause male pattern baldness – loss of hair at the temples and crown of your head. And without enough estrogen to stimulate your hair follicles, you're going to see generalized thinning of your hair.

Hair follicles need estrogen and thyroid hormone, particularly T_3, to grow. Estrogen affects how long the hair stays in certain stages. The hair on your head is in one of three stages. A growing stage, a stagnant stage, and a shedding stage. During the change, hair will be in the stagnant stage for longer periods of time. With less estrogen, there's less active growth. While hair density thins with age, low estrogen levels in menopause accelerates hair loss.

Another common dermatosis of menopause is the thickening of the soles of your feet and the palms of your hands. The soles of your feet can become calloused, cracked, and dry, due to the lack of estrogen.

Thickening is not limited to your feet and hands. Vulvar lichen sclerosus – thick white patches on the vulva that are not yeast infections – becomes very common due to low estrogen tissue levels. If not treated, lichen sclerosis can cause incredible pain and scarring. Strange pain sensations in your vulva and vagina, called dysesthetic vulvodynia, can also occur due to the nerves being affected by the lack of estrogen.

Without adequate estrogen, you're at increased risk for getting vaginal yeast infections. Healthy vaginal flora – lactobacillus acidophilus – helps protect you from Candida overgrowth. The pH of the vagina should be very acidic, about 4.6 or lower. Without adequate estrogen, vaginal pH rises, becoming alkaline, which is not a favorable environment for lactobacillus acidophilus to protect you.

Vaginal atrophy, or severe thinning of the vaginal tissues, happens to about 50% of postmenopausal women. Only 20% if they're taking systemic hormone replacement therapy, but some women still need topical vaginal estrogen to heal their vaginas.

Atrophic vulvovaginitis is characterized by dryness, irritation, soreness, pain during intercourse, increased urinary frequency, urgency, and urge incontinence. Your bladder and urethra are also estrogen dependent, so without adequate estrogen, you feel like you have to urinate all the time.

Periodontal disease becomes much more common in menopause. When women come to me for their consults, I do a complete physical, head to toe. I can see their receding gums when their estrogen levels are off, and ask what kind of dental work they've had done in the last few years.

Often they'll say, "I've had to have cavities refilled. I've had crowns that have become loose. I'm having issues with my gums; they bleed more easily. I'm having to get my teeth cleaned more often." It's because estrogen keeps your gums nice and lush and healthy.

During pregnancy, it's common to see almost an overgrowth of gum tissue due to very high estrogen levels. Just like the vulva and the vagina get swollen, so do the gums. When you go through menopause and postmenopause, your gums start to recede. If your gums recede enough, the roots of your teeth become exposed, and can get infected. You can actually lose your teeth due to low hormone levels.

Progesterone is also important for healthy gums, because it stimulates inflammatory mediators. When your progesterone levels fall in perimenopause, you are more likely to have inflammation of your gums, as well as more cavities and infections.

The microorganisms in your mouth are needed to synthesize enzymes that actually help with your hormone synthesis and detoxification. Your hormones help to keep your mouth bacteria healthy, and your oral flora keeps your hormones healthy. It's a symbiotic relationship.

Loss of breast fullness is very common in menopausal women. Estrogen and progesterone stimulate the mammary gland, the fibers in the breast, and even the fat that fills up most of our breast tissue. As your hormones decline, your breasts seem less full, and a little more saggy.

Your skin can become very, very itchy. There's two connections there. One is because your skin is dry, due to lack of estrogen. The other is because you tend to have strange cortisol reactions when you're menopausal. If you start scratching, you're going to have a rash, but it's usually itching without a rash until you start irritating your skin. And it can happen anywhere in your body – your scalp, your chest, your belly, or your back.

Menopausal pruritus is usually in the same spot, but the itching can spread. This is due to your cortisol being off its normal circadian pattern, because your hypothalamus is hyper-stimulating your adrenals to make cortisol at strange times.

Wrinkles are probably the most expected skin change. In menopause, you have decreased collagen content. Collagen is the protein-like tissue that holds your skin together. It holds your skin to your muscles, and your muscles to your bone. Estrogen helps stimulate healthy collagen production, but due to lack of estrogen, your skin becomes thin and wrinkled.

Decreased androgens in postmenopause lead to skin sagging. That's because testosterone helps hold your skin to your muscles, and mainly keeps your muscles stronger, bulks them up, and gives some surface area to your skin. Without testosterone in the post-menopausal phase, you're going to see more changes in your skin, like crepiness, which is fine dry wrinkling, mostly on your legs and arms.

Your hormones affect blood flow to the skin, which means without adequate estrogen, progesterone, and testosterone, your skin doesn't get enough oxygen, nutrition, or fluid .

As your hormone levels fall, you're going to notice that you might have less pubic and armpit hair. Now, that may not be a bad thing, but that is a clear sign that your hormone levels have fallen.

What I see in women who've gone through the second menopause, where their adrenals are really low-functioning, is that they often have very patchy pubic hair. This is because their DHEA levels are low as well. DHEA stimulates pubic hair growth in puberty, and when your adrenals poop out in postmenopause, you lose pubic hair.

You may notice that fine vellus hair on your head has been replaced by thick coarse hair, which is an androgen effect. In menopause, you have more male hormones on board than female hormones, which changes the texture of your hair.

Body odor is one of those symptoms that many postmenopausal and menopausal women will notice, but few talk about. Body odor is caused by androgen dominance, because as your estrogen levels fall, you have more testosterone floating around.

Testosterone stimulates sebum, which is an oil produced by skin cells that causes comedones or blackheads. Sebum feeds the bacteria in your skin, armpits, groin, and feet, so you'll notice more body odor.

Now, let's talk about skin tags. Skin tags are little protuberances of tissue that literally look like a tag on your shirt. Skin tags are common around your neck, underneath your breasts, and in your armpits. They tend to be in areas that might get irritated by collars, necklaces, your bra, or by shaving under your armpit.

Skin tags commonly develop in the perimenopausal period when you don't have enough progesterone to protect you from abnormal growth. Remember, progesterone is the gardener that tells estrogen to stop fertilizing growth. Skin tags are the result of estrogen fertilizing the weeds with not enough progesterone to calm them down. By postmenopause, fewer skin tags develop, but that doesn't mean they fall off. They will have to be removed, either by cutting or freezing them off.

Your nails can become very brittle, starting in perimenopause and continuing through postmenopause. Without adequate estrogen, you lose calcium from your nails as well as your bones.

Osteoporosis is a big problem associated with the change. One out of three women in her fifties suffers from bone loss. Osteopenia is mild bone loss, while osteoporosis means you've lost enough bone to have a high risk of fracture, usually in your hips or spine.

Bone loss begins when your estrogen levels fall, and without adequate progesterone, testosterone, growth hormone, and DHEA, you're not able to build bone as fast as you're losing it.

It's natural to get rid of all the old calcium and minerals in your bones and restructure it. In fact, you literally build an entire new skeleton every 12 to 18 months. However, if your bone loss is greater than your ability to build it back, you're going to develop osteoporosis.

Your posture can become adversely affected by bone loss. Osteoporosis of your vertebrae can cause your spine to curve, creating a dowager's hump at the top of your shoulders. Your head appears to be jutting forward, and your shoulders are humped.

Just as you're losing bone mass, you can lose muscle mass during the change. Muscle atrophy in postmenopause leads to weakness and poor balance, contributing to falls. Muscles need adequate testosterone, DHEA, and growth hormone to maintain strength and volume. Loss of lean body mass, including muscle and bone, contributes to lower metabolism and increase in body fat.

Ligaments and tendons can become stiff with lack of estrogen. Stiff ligaments affect joint function, and stiff tendons affect muscle function. Hormones help to keep your connective tissue flexible.

Vision changes are also common. In perimenopause, you may start noticing that you have what I call "short arm syndrome," meaning you're no longer able to see things close up. You start needing reading glasses.

You may wonder why this is happening. The menopausal loss of collagen causes your eyeball to change shape, which affects your vision. Besides stimulating collagen production, estrogen also stimulates fluid in all of your cells, including the vitreous fluid of your eyes. The fluid inside the eye affects the pressure of the eye. The fluid is controlled by little gateways, which become stiff from the lack of estrogen, increasing the pressure in your eye. Increased ocular pressure can lead to glaucoma.

Postmenopausal women have lower contrast sensitivity detection, meaning that it's harder for them to see in certain lights, as well as different colors and shadowing. That's why the first thing to go is your night vision. You start needing more light to read. All of this is because your hormones are lower.

Your cornea actually changes shape, so if you were able to use contact lenses to help your vision, you may find that they don't fit any longer once you're menopausal. One of the interesting things that I have seen by supporting your hypothalamus is that your cornea can retain a much more youthful shape, preserving your vision longer.

At 60, I'm really fortunate that I don't need to wear reading glasses. I believe this is because I've supported my hypothalamus since I was premenopausal.

Neurological Responses to the Change

Your neurological system also responds to the change, or lack of hormones. Clinical observations suggest your hormonal status affects your central and peripheral nervous systems.

Hormones affect your senses, your hearing, your sense of taste, and your sense of smell, but they also affect your entire nervous system. Estrogen helps your nerves to fire faster, while progesterone helps to myelinate the sheath, or the insulation around the nerve, keeping the nerve impulses on track.

Headaches are the most common neurological symptom. Migraines tend to be induced by a drop in estrogen, which is why we see premenstrual and menstrual migraines. When your estrogen drops to its lowest, it can trigger a vascular spasm.

While premenopausal migraines will eventually improve after menopause, during perimenopause, migraines can get worse because hormones are all over the place. If you've had a surgical menopause, meaning that your ovaries were removed along with your uterus, the drop in hormones is so drastic that your migraines can get much worse. Tension headaches are common in menopause because of increased muscle tension and nerve sensitivity.

Burning mouth syndrome is a neurological condition where the inside of your mouth and tongue become incredibly painful, causing a burning-like sensation. Burning mouth syndrome is a neural dysregulation of pain stimuli. Your nerves react as if you drank scalding hot liquid because you don't have enough estrogen on board to properly fire your nerves, nor enough progesterone to insulate your nerves to prevent misfiring. Burning mouth syndrome is very common in postmenopausal women with up to 30% prevalence, and it can start as early as perimenopause.

Fifty percent of menopausal women complain of arthralgia, or joint pain. Menopause can trigger swollen, stiff painful joints, and any joint can be affected – vertebrae in your back, hips, knees, neck, shoulders, jaw, elbows, and hands. Menopausal joint pain tends to affect joints that have been overused. So if you were a runner, and you have wear and tear on your knees, they may not bother you until perimenopause or menopause.

Once I reached menopause, running really aggravated my knees. I was a long distance runner and triathlete for decades, so I put a lot of miles on my knees.

If you did a lot of typing, you may have a little bit of joint damage in your hands and wrists that didn't bother you when you were younger, but now that you're going through menopause, you have more inflammation in your joints.

Your sex steroids affect your inflammatory mediators. If you don't have enough progesterone and estrogen to calm down the inflammatory mediators, you're going to have more joint pain.

The more menopausal symptoms a woman suffers, the more likely she will experience muscle pain and tension. Meaning, if she has a lot of hot flashes, insomnia, vaginal dryness, or any of the low hormone symptoms, she's going to notice that she has a lot more muscle pain, tension, and stiffness.

Breast soreness affects many women going through the change. It gets worse in early perimenopause and calms down in late perimenopause. This is because you're estrogen dominant in early perimenopause, and you become less estrogen dominant as you progress towards menopause. So you're not getting as much stimulation of your breasts, and they won't be quite as swollen, sensitive, or tender.

Progesterone can also aggravate breast tenderness, so you've got to be careful with hormone replacement therapy. For some women, estrogen therapy can actually increase breast pain. While breast pain is very common throughout perimenopause, it usually does not extend into postmenopause.

You may notice strange nerve sensations. Hormone levels affect your central nervous system, and when estrogen and progesterone start to fluctuate, your nerves are impacted. The strange nerve sensations during the change can take the form of tingling and burning, or can create a sense that your skin is crawling.

You might feel cold, numbness, a pins and needles sensation, and increased sensitivity. Because of the lack of progesterone, you don't have proper myelin sheath laid down, so your nerves are misfiring.

And the lack of estrogen prevents nerve messages from getting to the central nervous system, so your brain can not interpret the sensations appropriately.

You can have tingling extremities. This is partly because low estrogen means lower collagen production, resulting in thinner skin and reduced blood flow to the nerves of your extremities. Additionally, progesterone is no longer laying down that healthy myelin, which also contributes to tingling.

You may notice an irregular heartbeat as early as perimenopause. Estrogen affects the way your heart beats by affecting serotonin production, not just in your brain, but in your heart. Your heart rhythm is controlled by a nerve bundle lying between the atrium and the ventricles called the AV node. Like all of your nerves, the AV node is affected by your hormones, so you might experience palpitations or a racing heart anytime throughout the change.

These heart palpitations are usually non-threatening arrhythmias, meaning they're not dangerous. You may go to a family doctor or a cardiologist to get them checked out. After vigorous diagnostic testing, you'll find that there's nothing cardiac-wise that's wrong. It's because your hormones are too low to properly fire the AV node that controls your heart rate.

Another neurological symptom is dizzy spells, called benign paroxysmal positional vertigo. When your head changes position from lying down to getting up, or turning over in bed, you can get short spells of vertigo or dizziness. This is because crystals in your cochlea, your inner ear, become dislodged. Positional vertigo is two times more common in women than in men. In perimenopause, estrogen affects the fluid levels in the inner ear, which can cause an increase in dizziness. Vertigo is much more common in menopausal women, and if you've had a premenopausal oophorectomy, meaning your ovaries were removed, vertigo becomes worse because you've lost your hormones too drastically.

You can also experience a change in your sense of smell. Hormones affect the airflow, the pressure in your nasal passages during respiration, as well as your olfactory nerves, or the nerves that pick up odor. Your sense of smell changes in response to where your hormones are.

Pregnant women can be particularly hypersensitive to odor. It's due to their high hormone levels. And it's not unusual in the preovulatory period of a reproductively viable woman for her to notice that her sense of smell is much more acute. Your sense of smell can actually be depressed by postmenopause, where you don't smell as acutely as you once did.

I've personally noticed that all through perimenopause and into early menopause, my sense of smell has been heightened. I can smell blooming jasmine acres away. No one else around me will smell it, yet if I follow my nose, I find it. It's like being a menopausal bloodhound. Nerves are funny, sometimes becoming less sensitive, other times more.

We know that olfactory nerves are affected by hormones because of a congenital condition called Kallmann syndrome. These people have hypogonadism, meaning their gonads aren't functioning properly with very little sex hormone production, and they also have no sense of smell.

Sex steroids affect olfactory perception within the brain. As an embryo, your sense of smell is laid down at the same time as the cells in your hypothalamus that affect ovarian production of hormones, particularly progesterone. When you go through menopause, your sense of smell is affected. And if your sense of smell is affected, so is your taste. Food just doesn't taste good anymore.

Since many of these lesser-known symptoms of the change affect our quality of life, it's important to be aware of them and get the help you need.

ACTION ~ What lesser-known symptoms are affecting you?

Lesser Known Symptoms

Hypothalamic responses to the Change	Digestive tract responses to the Change	Dermatological and Connective tissue responses to the Change	Nervous system responses to the Change
Hot flashes	Digestive problems	Vaginal dryness	Headaches
Insomnia	Nausea	Gum problems	Burning mouth
Weight gain	Constipation	Loss of breast fullness	Joint pain
Mood swings	Bloating	Itchy skin	Breast soreness
Low sex drive		Rashes	Electric shocks
Night sweats		Wrinkles	Muscle tension
Irregular periods		Skin tags	Tingling extremities
Fatigue		Brittle nails	Irregular heartbeat
Anxiety		Hair loss	Dizzy spells
Memory lapses		Stress incontinence	
Difficulty concentrating		Osteoporosis	
Irritability			
Depression			
Panic disorder			
Allergies			
Vulnerability to infections			
Body odor			

© D Maragopoulos 2021

Chapter 6

Your Risk Factors

Five years after having a radical mastectomy and radiation for invasive breast cancer, Karen consults with me. She's exhausted all the time, can't sleep, has absolutely no sex drive, and her vagina is so dry that intercourse is impossible. A health and fitness nut, in spite of her best efforts, she's gained ten pounds. She has horrible brain fog which is preventing her from doing her job. In spite of the risks of a recurrent cancer, Karen swears she can't live like this anymore. "Please, please, give me some hormones," she begs.

Cancer cannot be taken lightly. And while Karen's breast cancer was successfully treated – her oncologists did not address the root cause – so there's always a chance it can reoccur. And exogenous estrogen can feed rogue cells.

So we begin with vaginal estriol – a safe treatment to offer women with estrogen dependent cancers, as vaginal absorption is low. But we don't stop there. Karen needs hormonal support. Vaginal estrogen will not help her brain fog, fatigue, or insomnia.

Evaluating her estrogen metabolism helps guide our treatment. Like most breast cancer patients, Karen's blood work reveals high conversion of estradiol to inflammatory and carcinogenic forms of estrone. So we begin helping her body metabolize estrogen more safely by increasing IC_3 indoles, fish oils, ipriflavone, and flax lignans in her diet, and by limiting alcohol and toxic exposures.

We also begin supporting her hypothalamus which effectively resets her day/night cycles, and she starts sleeping through the night. Her energy increases and her memory improves. Then, we add appropriate hormones that her body had been deficient in, and follow up with estrogen metabolism tests to be sure she metabolizes her hormones safely.

The point of this chapter is for you to better understand what you need to know about yourself to make the safest choices during menopause.

Every woman has to consider her personal risk factors, and weigh them against the quality of her life with and without hormones. It's an individual choice, but first you need to know your risk factors.

When a patient comes to see me and I suspect that she's perimenopausal or even menopausal, I am definitely going to take a full history, including asking about her physical symptoms, her personal history, her sexual history, her spiritual life, everything she's ever done to her body and in her life that may affect her hormones. Before we do any blood work, before I do a physical examination, before we make any decisions on treatment, I need to know who she is as a person, and who she was hormonally when she was younger, so I can figure out how out of balance she is now, and what types of treatment would be the safest for her.

So let's talk about the risk factors that might affect your change of life, whether you're premenopausal, perimenopausal, menopausal, or postmenopausal.

We think of risk factors just being for treatment, used to determine whether or not it's safe and appropriate to offer you hormones, but there are also risk factors of not having hormones. You'll want to consider what's going to happen to you when you go through the change because your hormones are depleted.

These risk factors have multiple layers, the first of which are your genetics.

Your Genetics

The first layer we're going to talk about is your genetics. This is something you can't control, right? Isn't DNA set in stone?

Well, not exactly. Only a small portion of your DNA is expressed. Most people don't realize that most of your genetics are not expressed.

Let's say we're playing a game of cards, and we each get seven cards. Those seven cards are what we have expressed – our physical appearance, our biochemical makeup, our biological function. Your seven cards are your expression and my seven cards are my expression. You also have a stack of cards next to you, which are unexpressed DNA. The expressed DNA is the color of your hair, skin and eyes, your body shape, your tendencies towards breast cancer, heart disease, diabetes, osteoporosis – that's all in your genetics.

The cards that you could borrow in that stack of unexpressed DNA can change the expressed DNA, and ultimately, the outcome of the game of life. You're not stuck with what you're born with, genetically speaking. The lifestyle choices you make, what you eat, how you deal with stress, the kind of environmental exposures you have, and how active you are all affect your genetics.

Genetic testing has become very popular. It can tell you what genes you have that may or may not express disease. Yet, science is not yet capable of interpreting the millions of genes in your DNA, so genetic testing only reveals a small aspect of your genetic potential.

I want you to understand that you have the power to change your DNA through your choices. Now, the choices you've already made have taken an effect, but you can reverse some of it.

Your Family History

While you have the power to change your genetic expression, you do need to be aware of the cards in your hand. And you need to make your health care provider aware of your family history. For example, if you have heart disease within your family, you may have some genetic propensity towards arteriosclerosis. There are genetic familial types of very high cholesterol. You need to know about that. If there are strokes or heart attacks in your family history, we need to know about that.

If there's an issue with diabetes in your family, particularly type 2 diabetes, we need to know. Type 1 diabetes is juvenile diabetes, and considered an autoimmune issue, but type 2 diabetes tends to run in families. If obesity runs in the family, especially obesity associated with type 2 diabetes, we need to know about that.

Is there cancer in your family? Have any of your maternal relatives had breast cancer, either pre or postmenopausal? Premenopausal breast cancer is much more aggressive than postmenopausal breast cancer, but it'll give us information about how safe it is for you to use hormones or not, as well as what kind of testing we can do to make sure it is safe for you. If there is breast cancer in the family, was it the BRCA gene, and have you been tested for that?

Is there colon cancer in the family? Colon cancer is also an estrogen related cancer, as is melanoma, a type of skin cancer that can happen when you're younger. Is there prostate cancer in the males of your family? There is a correlation between familial prostate cancer and women developing gynecological cancers, such as ovarian and uterus cancers. Is there Alzheimer's or dementia in the family? Does osteoporosis run in your family?

Your family's lifestyle is really what's going to turn on those genes. For instance, if your mother has osteoporosis, but she was a smoker and a drinker, and you're not, you have less likelihood of developing osteoporosis. If she didn't exercise at all and you do, you have less likelihood of developing the disease. Your genetic expression is affected by the choices you make and the behaviors you carry out.

There are other things to consider when you go through the change, such as when your mother went through menopause. Did she suffer badly from symptoms? Some women, especially in my generation, may not really know what happened with their mothers, because moms didn't talk about it. So you may not have much of that information, but if you do, whether it's a mother, a grandmother, an aunt, even an older sister, that would be good to know. If your mother or any of your maternal relatives have diseases like diabetes, heart disease, stroke, or any cancers that they developed in postmenopause, we want to know.

Your Personal History

Your personal history, meaning your gynecological and medical history, is different from your family history.

When did you start your periods? We know that women who started their periods before the age of 12 have a slightly higher risk of developing estrogen-related cancers, because they usually have their periods for a lot longer. Or if they go through menopause late, like after the age of 55, then they're exposed to endogenous (their own) estrogen longer. There may be a slightly increased risk for breast cancer, ovarian cancer, uterine cancer, or endometrial cancer.

Your Risk Factors 75

Were your periods regular? I know it seems crazy that we're talking about regularity, when your periods may have stopped altogether, but a lot of women continue to cycle just like they did when they were younger, even though they may not get a period to show for it.

I'd like to know how many days your cycles lasted, and if you followed the moon cycle. It gives me more information to work with if we do start hormone replacement therapy, and allows us to schedule days off of the hormones to mimic your natural cycles.

Did you have a lot of pain with your periods? Did you have heavy bleeding? Did you have issues with endometriosis? Fibroids? Cysts? What was your PMS like? This information indicates how sensitive you are to your hormones plummeting. What kinds of symptoms did you get premenstrually? Was it breast tenderness or bloating? Were you super moody? Did you have premenstrual dysphoria, or severe premenstrual depression, almost a psychosis? How you reacted to your hormonal fluctuations then will affect how you're reacting to them now.

What was your birth control history? Did you use any birth control that was hormonal, such as oral birth control pills, shots, vaginal rings, or implants? Different hormonal birth control methods can adversely affect your hypothalamus.

Research shows that the hypothalamus actually shrinks by 5% in women who take the birth control pill (BCP), especially for a prolonged period of time. I've seen issues with hypothalamic dysfunction in women who have taken the birth control pill for less than two years. So we need to know if you've been on hormonal contraceptives to get an idea of how healthy your hypothalamus is coming into the change.

What was your response to the hormonal contraceptive? Did you have side effects during or after stopping it? Perhaps you were fine while on BCPs, but afterwards you broke out like crazy because your testosterone was a little high.

Did you have a tubal ligation? Research shows that women who've had their tubes tied suffer from more hot flashes. When I was working with a gynecologist, I noticed that our patients who had any type of surgical manipulation of their ovaries or Fallopian tubes, including tubal ligation, seemed to have hormonal imbalances afterwards. The surgeon didn't want to believe my anecdotal findings until I discovered a study that showed that after tubal ligation, women had lower progesterone levels. Since the Fallopian tubes are part of the hormonal communication network between the ovaries and the hypothalamus, any disruption like a tubal ligation may cause hormone imbalances.

We need to know if you've ever been pregnant. In terms of estrogen-related cancers, pregnancy can be protective. They're most protective when you have pregnancies between the ages of 15 and 25. Yet pregnancy at any time in life is protective. Breastfeeding also provides some protection in terms of estrogen-related cancers, especially of the breast. Yet some pregnancy complications can make you more prone to postmenopausal issues. If you had pre-eclampsia, you may have an increased risk for heart disease and stroke when you become menopausal. If you suffered from postpartum depression, you have an increased risk of menopausal depression.

We also need to know if you have had infertility treatment, especially multiple treatments, because that exogenous (not your own) hormone exposure can increase your risk for ovarian cancer, even later in life. Hormonal infertility treatments can also cause issues with your hypothalamus.

If you had fibroids when you were younger and going into menopause, you may have noticed those fibroids getting bigger and bigger. And then postmenopausally, they'll shrink. Did you have ovarian cysts? Were you a heavy bleeder? Maybe you had adenomyosis, which is a cystic condition of the lining of the uterus, causing incredibly heavy bleeding, almost hemorrhagic. Oftentimes, women with adenomyosis will have uterine ablation with hot saline, or even electrolysis to burn off their uterine lining. But these treatments don't always work to stop their hemorrhagic periods.

Were you diagnosed with endometriosis? Most of these conditions – fibroids, cysts, the heavy bleeding of adenomyosis, and endometriosis – all get better after menopause. Not having your hormones anymore actually improves all those gynecological conditions, but perimenopause can be a bear because your hormones are all over the place. Because of this, we have to be aware and help you through those changes.

And finally, we must consider what environmental exposures you've had. Meaning, in your work environment, home environment, or where you grew up, were there any toxins? Heavy metals, plastic exposures, xenoestrogens? Any type of environmental exposures that would increase your risk for certain cancers or certain auto-immune diseases? All of these things are going to be exacerbated in menopause because your immune system is affected by your low hormones. So whatever you have circulating in your system, or even hidden in your system, like lead in your bones, can actually become an issue later when your immune system can't fight it off anymore.

Your Lifestyle

Your risk factors are definitely influenced by your lifestyle. Have you been active throughout your life, or were you very sedentary? Did you have a sitting job? Were you athletic? We now know that being sedentary, meaning that you sit most of the time and are not very active at all, is just as dangerous as smoking in terms of heart disease and metabolic diseases.

What has your nutrition been like throughout your life? Did you grow up on a Standard American Diet, also known as SAD – high fat, particularly trans fats, lots of processed foods and sugars? If so, this can be a huge issue coming into menopause.

Were you vegan? Vegans may have issues coming into menopause because of their high exposure to soy proteins. Soy blocks T_3 activity and estrogen receptors. Were you like my generation, growing up on low fat and artificial sweeteners? Consuming these does not provide a great foundation for coming into menopause. You're nutritionally deficient to start with. Perhaps you didn't have the healthiest diet in your youth, but in the past 10 years, you've cleaned up your act. That's great, but I still want to know where you came from so we can see what your foundation was built on.

What chemical exposures have you had? Tobacco, alcohol, recreational drugs, and over-the-counter or prescription medications all count. One-time exposure is not an issue, but multiple exposures to anything stimulating or sedating, we need to know about. Medications for adult hyperactivity disorder, antidepressants, anti-anxiety medications, anything that you've been taking for a long period of time can affect the way your brain and body are functioning, and you're going to have a different foundation than an unmedicated woman coming into menopause. Any supplements you're taking – especially high doses for extended periods of time, makes me wonder what you've been self-treating.

What is your marital status? Yes, whether you're single, divorced, or married affects your experience in menopause. Studies show that married women generally go through menopause a little later. Other factors include how many children you've had, as well as your income 10 years prior to menopause. The decade prior to the change of life affects your experience of menopause, based on how much stress you've been under. Maybe you've been stressed by financial concerns, an unhappy relationship, the loss of loved ones, the loss of a job, divorce, or remarriage and combining families. What you've had to live through in the decade before menopause highly affects your experience.

Studies show that women in unsatisfying marriages report increased stress and far more menopausal symptoms than women who have satisfying marriages. Satisfaction was measured by self report of adequate social support, good communication, and sexual satisfaction. What's happening in your life really does make a difference. Your relationships affect how you're experiencing the change, because hormones are messengers. And when you get into better balance, it positively affects your relationships.

So many times over the years, I've consulted with a menopausal woman, and as soon as we get her in balance, she brings in her husband because he's also going through his own change, called andropause. Our hormones affect one another.

Do you have dependents, whether they're children, adult children dependent on you, grandchildren dependent on you, or parents who are dependent on you? Taking care of others affects your experience in menopause. If you don't have time to take care of yourself, you're going to have a lot more symptoms and not be as healthy. Do you have issues with codependency, in which you have trouble letting go and not taking care of yourself? This is important to know about yourself going into the change, so that you can start prioritizing your own health.

I'm not saying that you have to stop helping your children, parents, or spouse, or that you're not going to do your best at your job. What I am saying is that if you have codependency issues and you have a tendency to prioritize yourself last, your menopause experience is going to be a lot harder. The change can be the perfect opportunity to start prioritizing your health and your well-being. You'll feel so much better about going through the change with your symptoms in control that you'll be at your best for everyone else in your life.

Do you have a high stress lifestyle? Are you traveling a lot? Have you been exposed to multiple stressors? Multiple losses, changes, and transitions are common in midlife. Divorces happen, deaths happen, and careers change. Maybe you're dealing with children getting married and grandbabies arriving. Maybe you're dealing with your parents getting older. Maybe your grandparents are dying.

So many things are happening at the same time you're going through the change. And all that progesterone that your ovaries were making to support your adrenal glands' production of stress hormones is not there anymore. Because of this, you're experiencing stress at a much higher level, which means it's affecting you physically, mentally, and emotionally.

Do you have comorbidities?

Comorbidities mean that you have other diagnoses besides being menopausal that can complicate the change of life. The majority of my patients have comorbidities, and very few consult with me just about menopause. They're also dealing with hypothyroid problems, their adrenals are out of balance, or they may already have been diagnosed with cancer, osteoporosis, heart disease, or autoimmunity. There have been a lot of studies on what happens in menopause when you have comorbidities, and also how menopause affects these diseases.

One of the biggest comorbidities coming into menopause is osteoporosis.

Osteoporosis affects about 10 million Americans, =80% of which are women. One in two women over the age of 50 will break a bone because of osteoporosis. The risk of breaking your hip is equal to your combined risk of breast, uterine, and ovarian cancer. We are so afraid of cancers, but osteoporosis is much more common and can make your life absolutely miserable. Coming into menopause with a low bone density to start with because you didn't eat well during your life, you weren't active, or you have genetic propensity towards osteoporosis is an issue. The risk rises with early menopause. If you go through menopause earlier, you're more likely to develop osteoporosis because you're without estrogen longer. If you did not breastfeed or didn't breastfeed for very long, or if you're a cigarette smoker, you're going to have a higher risk for osteoporosis.

However, cardiovascular disease is the big killer. Your cardiovascular system is affected by estrogen. As your estrogen levels lower, it increases the risk of metabolic dysfunction, which is the inflammation of your arteries, and increases your risk of heart attack and stroke. When you go through menopause, the type of cholesterol you make changes. Most pre-menopausal women have healthy cholesterol profiles. They make lots of protective HDL, and their LDL particles tend to be big, buoyant, and protective. But once they go through the change, they make much less HDL, they have higher levels of triglycerides, which increases their risk of arteriosclerosis, and their LDL cholesterol molecules are smaller, denser, and more likely to cause plaque, which contributes to strokes and heart attacks.

If you come into menopause and you're already diabetic, especially if you have type 2 diabetes, you have an increased risk of metabolic issues. Metabolic issues are inflammatory conditions that include insulin resistance, obesity, high blood pressure, and high cholesterol. All of those things together are part of metabolic syndrome. I check all my patients for metabolic markers, because these are the big killers. It's really important we get this under control and take your metabolic condition into consideration when we're offering you therapy.

What about other inflammatory diseases? Perimenopause is a proinflammatory state, especially for the neurological system. Estrogen is a master regulator that controls the neurotransmitter receptors in your brain. Estradiol also helps stimulate neurological plasticity, meaning the neurons actually learn, grow, and adapt to preserve your health and wellbeing.

Progesterone helps to myelinate neuron sheaths, so that the nervous impulses can get where they're going as quickly as possible. When your estrogen and progesterone levels are falling in perimenopause, you start to have inflammation in your nervous system, especially in your brain. Estrogen regulates mitochondrial function, or your ability to produce energy. Low estrogen is one of the reasons why we see a lot more brain fog when you're going through the change.

Inflammatory diseases like arthritis can also be affected by the change. Remember, autoimmune diseases may become worse, as can asthma and pulmonary issues.

If you come into menopause and you've already been diagnosed with cancer, it may affect treatment options. There's a particular concern regarding breast cancer. If you've experienced a late menopause after the age of 55, or you started menstruating before the age of 12, you may have an increased risk for breast cancer, as well as ovarian and uterine cancers. Long exposure to your natural estrogens, xenoestrogens in the environment, or \added estrogen through birth control pills or infertility treatments can increase the risk of estrogen-related cancers.

Colon cancer is usually not picked up until your 50's, but it isn't highly unusual for me to see patients in their late 30's and 40's with colon cancer. A prospective study of over 55,000 women found that those who took menopausal hormone replacement therapy had a reduced risk of colorectal cancer. Hormones are beneficial for your colon, but every woman needs to take all of her risk factors into consideration.

So, what about skin cancer? The risk is about the same if you use hormone replacement or you don't. If you have a history of melanoma, or if it runs in the family, we worry about hormone replacement therapy, because estrogen stimulates the melanocytes. But we don't have to worry about hormone replacement therapy if you have sun-related skin cancers.

What if you're coming into menopause with early signs of dementia? Estrogen influences the function of your brain in areas that are related to learning and retrieving information, especially for language and judgment. When your estrogen is gone, you lose dendritic cells, which are the little tiny nerve hairs that allow the nerves to talk to one another.

You lose the synapses – the communication network – which is why you start missing information and memory. You're going to see a lot more issues with your cognition and your mood. Women who have more vasovagal responses in perimenopause like hot flashes tend to experience a worsening of their memory. These women are really sensitive to estrogen falling.

Dementia can also be caused by vascular issues. Estrogen affects the health of arteries, and as estrogen levels fall, increasing inflammation leads to arteriosclerosis. Low blood flow due to micro-hemorrhages (small bleeds in the brain) and transient ischemic attacks (mini strokes) are much more common causes of dementia than Alzheimer's.

The metabolic changes in the brain that happen in menopause can increase the risk of Alzheimer's disease. That's why we see more women with Alzheimer's disease than men. Lower estrogen at mid-life contributes to late onset Alzheimer's. However, this doesn't mean every woman going through menopause is going to develop Alzheimer's. If you have a family history of Alzheimer's disease, there is genetic testing that can be done to determine whether or not you may be prone to Alzheimer's.

If you have a dual diagnosis, meaning you're going through menopause and you also have hypothyroidism, diabetes, cancer, autoimmunity, a pituitary tumor, central obesity, heart disease, metabolic syndrome, or insulin resistance, menopause is going to be more complicated. We have to be really sure we're giving you the right therapy, because sometimes it can help, while other times, it can make your condition worse.

You want to be sure that you're treating menopause symptoms, not just assuming this is the other disease. For instance, hypothyroidism can be worse when you go through menopause because estrogen helps to upregulate your T3 receptors. So it can't just be assumed that your thyroid levels are dropping just because you're getting older. It could be the change that will settle once you become postmenopausal, but the hormonal rollercoaster of perimenopause and menopause is making that worse now.

The same goes for hypertension, and even your cholesterol can be affected by menopause. Your cholesterol naturally rises when you go through the change, because you need more of the big buoyant LDL cholesterol to make estrogen, progesterone, and testosterone. Because of this expected rise, I measure cholesterol sub-particles, not just total cholesterol levels. That way, we can see if we're treating a hormone issue versus a metabolic issue.

What if you have polycystic ovary syndrome (PCOS)? If you have polycystic ovary syndrome, you may go through menopause a little bit earlier. Now, PCOS is a hyperandrogenic disorder, meaning you make too much male hormone. It's the most common endocrinopathy issue of premenopausal women. When you have PCOS, you're more likely to have fertility issues because you don't ovulate regularly. Because you have too much testosterone onboard, you may have hairiness, central obesity, insulin resistance, inflammation, and metabolic disturbances. Fortunately, PCOS gets better once you go through the change, but if you have not controlled your PCOS, or if you have not treated the metabolic issues, not lost the weight, not become active, and not gotten those inflammatory markers down, menopause is going to make your metabolic issues worse.

We want to make sure that your PCOS is under control when you're premenopausal. I've had patients whose PCOS reversed with hypothalamic support, so they were able to get pregnant if they chose. This is because PCOS is not an ovarian issue, it's a hypothalamic issue. If you support your hypothalamus, menopause is so much easier.

Another comorbidity that is affected by the change is chronic fatigue syndrome. Women with chronic fatigue syndrome (CFS) are 12 times more likely to have pelvic pain, excessive bleeding and more bleeding between periods, more irregularity of their periods, and are more likely to use hormones like birth control to treat their symptoms. And they're more likely to have gynecological surgeries, particularly hysterectomy, than women who haven't had CFS. Chronic fatigue syndrome can complicate menopause, and going through menopause makes chronic fatigue symptoms worse. However, treating menopausal symptoms can make chronic fatigue symptoms much better.

Your Personal Assessment

When a woman going through the change consults with me, I don't just ask her about her family history, her genetics, her comorbidities, and her lifestyle, but I also observe her body type. By the time I see her, her body may have changed, she may have gained some weight, and she may have lost some muscle tone, yet her body type is still evident.

What kind of figure did you have in your younger years?

Did you have an estrogenic figure with curves – a small waist, carrying most of your body fat in your breasts, hips, and thighs? Did you have an androgenic figure – lean, athletic, muscular? Or did you have a cortisol driven figure – apple shaped and carrying weight in your abdomen with thin legs?

How you carry body fat, your natural musculature, and the thickness of your bones tells me what kind of hormones your body is used to. The estrogenic body type with the hourglass figure needs more estrogen. The more athletic body type can deal with less estrogen, a little bit of progesterone, and oftentimes likes a little testosterone. The woman who has more belly fat is often cortisol-dependent, and needs to have her insulin resistance addressed to prevent further weight gain. We want to definitely make sure she has enough estrogen and progesterone to control symptoms and prevent bone loss, but not give her too much testosterone because that'll increase her risk for metabolic issues.

I also like to talk to women about their sex life. Why? Because your sex life is going to change in menopause. And I want to prepare you for that. No matter how you've experienced sex in the past, there are going to be changes because your body has changed.

Sex can actually be amazing after menopause, but only if you're prepared. We discuss at length how to keep your vagina healthy. We also address your biggest sexual organ – your mind – so it's on board with having an active and pleasing sex life. If a woman is celibate or in between relationships, we still want to get her vagina as healthy as possible. Maybe she's not planning on having sex now, but we never know what might be coming up in the future. Also, a well estrogenized vagina helps support her urinary health.

I also like to look at your belief systems. There's been quite a bit of research comparing women who have a miserable menopause with women who have an empowered menopause. These two types of women have totally different belief systems when it comes to their health, their wellbeing, their sense of being a woman, and the change of life.

Women who are miserable in menopause assume that their worth is related to their youth. They do not see the value in aging and it's not their fault. Society sets us up to adore youth, and does not prefer older women or see them as beautiful, sexy, wise, and valuable.

Yet in reality, aged women are the gifts of our human existence. There are very few species of animals on the earth that have animals old enough to be considered grandmothers. Whales are one, and elephants are another. Biologists note that in whale and elephant families, having older females that are no longer reproductive within the group is protective for the entire group. It helps the babies and teenagers grow, and it protects the rest of the mothers in the group. The grandmothers pass on their survival knowledge to their pod or herd.

There is great value in having lived long enough to reach menopause. You have the wisdom gained from surviving this life that can be passed on to the next generation. Women tend to live longer than men because there is a biological value to us sticking around for the species.

So let's make this positive. The way we make the change of life positive is by being as empowered as possible, and being prepared for menopause. If you're prepared, educated and have a plan – a Menopause Action Plan – you won't look back at your youth and say, "Well, that was the best time." Today is the best day. And the future will be even better. It's all about your outlook.

I have seen women who look and act incredibly youthful. Yes, they're old chronologically, but their biology seems to be fairly young because they just don't believe in aging. They keep on with their life, and keep going and being as active as possible. They don't assume they can't do anything, or that they're now limited by their age. They start a whole new life after the change, a new career, new relationship, new hobbies, and a new outlook.

This is a new chapter of your life. And your belief systems will really guide you through the change. Even if you grew up in a family where all the women thought menopause was going to be miserable and it was miserable for them, you can change your personal belief system. It's up to you.

You may need some therapy, you may need some deprogramming, you may need to take some self-help courses and go to women's retreats. But you can change, if you desire to be empowered.

Empowered menopause means living your best life as a menopausal woman in all aspects – physically, emotionally, mentally, sexually, spiritually.

This leads to the very last piece that I want to look at when I'm assessing a woman going through the change. What is your spiritual life like? What was it in the past? And how has it shifted throughout your life?

I find women going through the change to be incredibly spiritually open. And I'm not talking about religion. I'm not talking about what you believe in, in terms of how you refer to the divine. I'm talking about being open to spirit. I'm talking about vibration and connection to everything in our life. Other people, animals, plants, and the Earth herself.

Women going through the change start to open up. Sometimes, that scares them. They start having dreams that are quite lucid and prolific – actually dreaming things before they happen. This type of dreaming happens for some women before menopause, but menopause can be a huge opening for others.

I believe we need to use this opening. This is our mystical potential, where menopause can be incredibly empowering. This can be an amazing journey, even more exciting than it was when you were younger, when all your intuition was used to survive your life, lead others, perhaps raise children. Now that's all done, your intuition can be used to actually guide every moment of being in this world, and menopause can be amazingly beautiful.

ACTION ~ What risk factors do you have that will influence how you will treat menopause?

Part Three

Connecting the Dots

Chapter 7

The Hypothalamic Connection

Your Hormones Sing and Your DNA Dances

Your Hypothalamus is the Maestro of Your Symphony of Hormones

If you were sitting with me in the office, we'd have already gone over your intake. We know where you are in the change of life, whether you're premenopausal, perimenopausal, menopausal, or post-menopausal. We've determined your risk factors. We've gone over all your history, your lifestyle, and your beliefs. Now it's time to teach you about your body and help you understand the connections.

This chapter focuses on the physical connections. And in the next, we're going to go into depth on the other connections – the psycho-spiritual, the vibrational, and all the things that your hormones are affecting outside of you.

Let's explore a more intimate perspective on how your internal physiology connects to your external reality. Albert Einstein demonstrated that matter and energy are interrelated. In fact, we have two types of medical philosophies in this world – energy-based medicine and matter-based medicine.

In matter-based medicine, or Western medicine, we usually don't believe something exists unless we can prove it with some kind of biological tool: a blood test, a urine test, or we can see it under a microscope. We need to be able to identify the matter. In energy-based medicine, which is considered Eastern, the assessments and treatments are based on energy. In the Eastern philosophy, you have seven power points in your body. They're called chakras, which translates to little wheels of energy.

In the Western point of view, those seven chakras are exactly where your endocrine glands lie, and where your hormones are produced. The first, or "root chakra," is where your gonads are. As women, that would be our ovaries. The second, or "navel chakra," corresponds to your pancreas. The third, "solar plexus chakra" corresponds to your adrenal glands. The fourth, "heart chakra" corresponds to your thymus. The fifth, "throat chakra" corresponds to your thyroid. Your pituitary gland is in the sixth "third eye chakra," while the seventh, "crown chakra" is your pineal gland.

East meets West, energy meets matter, in your endocrine system.

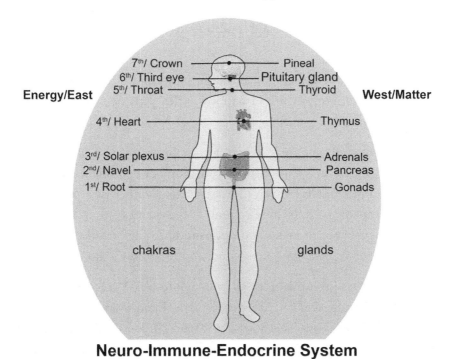

Neuro-Immune-Endocrine System

© D Maragopoulos 2021

I like to include the neurological and immune systems in there as well, because they all produce hormones. Now, hormone basically means messenger. The hormones of the seven endocrine glands are very big, while the hormones of the neurological system, the neurotransmitters, are just a little bit smaller. You know them as serotonin and dopamine, acetylcholine, GABA, and glutamate. They're messengers as well. And the hormones of the immune system, called cytokines, are little tiny cell messengers like interferon and interleukin.

All of these messenger "hormones" of your neuro-immune-endocrine system communicate what's going on between the energy and matter, both within and outside of your body. For instance, an apple tree converts sunlight (energy) into fruit (matter). The hormone insulin escorts the sugar from the apple into your cells, which they use to create energy.

While your endocrine system is vitally important, it does not work alone. Your hormones work in harmony with your neurological and immune systems.

Your neurological system is not just your brain; it's also your heart and your gut. In fact, your heart is your number one brain, meaning the most important for survival. Your gut is number two, and your brain is number three. If there's a limit to the quantity of amino acids you have available to make neurotransmitters, your heart's going to get the resources first, your gut second, and then your brain.

Your immune system includes all your white blood cells, which act like soldiers protecting you. It includes your thymus, which programs those soldiers to know exactly what to attack. If your immune system goes after you, that's called autoimmunity. Your tonsils, adenoids, appendix, as well as your lymph system, are part of your immune system. And your spleen recycles blood cells after retrieving information from your white blood cells to tell your thymus, via hormones, what's happening in your body, and what they should be going after.

Hormones are at work all the time, whether they're the traditional hormones like estrogen, progesterone, testosterone, or they're neurotransmitters or cytokines. But what actually controls all those hormones?

Think of all of the hormones in the neuro-immune-endocrine system as software programs for the hard drive of the body. You can't use a computer without software, and you cannot run the software without an operating system.

Your hypothalamus is your body's operating system.

Your hypothalamus is located just above the pituitary gland in the center of your brain. Super important and very much ignored in medicine, your hypothalamus controls every aspect of your vital systems. I believe it's in the center of your pyramid of health. Your pyramid of health is based on what's happening with your hormones. At the base of the pyramid are the hormones made from your ovaries. They keep you supported when you're young. When you go through the change of life, your base becomes narrower and you don't have all the support you used to have.

From your ovaries to your pancreas, your adrenals, your thymus, your thyroid, your pituitary and pineal gland, what runs your entire endocrine system is your hypothalamus.

Your hypothalamus is not protected by the blood-brain barrier. It knows exactly what's coming into the body, and it directs what goes out of the body. Nutrition and detoxification are two of the cornerstones on your pyramid of health.

By directing hormones, your hypothalamus talks to your DNA.

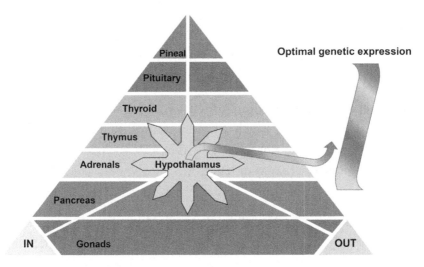

Hormones in Harmony

© D Maragopoulos 2021

Your genes express what the hypothalamus tells them to express. If you're expressing disease, it's because your hypothalamus is telling it to do so. It may look like a survival technique. For instance, insulin resistance has certain genes that get turned on due to a person's lifestyle. What they're eating, how active they are, if they're sleeping enough, how much stress they're under – when all of those conditions are poor, your hypothalamus helps you store extra calories in your belly fat to help you survive what it perceives as poor environmental conditions.

In nature, if you were a bear, your hypothalamus would turn on the same genes to prepare your body to hibernate for the winter, so you could live off that extra fat. Early humans would gain fat through the summer to hold them out through the winter when food was limited. Insulin resistance is part of natural survival genetics.

In modern times, however, winter doesn't prevent us from accessing food. If you're eating more calories than you're expending, you will become obese. That extra fat is being stored in your liver and around your organs, which is dangerous. If you were living in a time where you needed to hibernate for the winter, insulin resistance would be an adaptive genetic expression. Now, it's maladaptive.

Your genes are just encoding for what your hypothalamus is experiencing in your world, which you can control. Remember, DNA is like playing cards. It's not necessarily the cards you're dealt –it's more important how you play your hand.

When I first rediscovered the hypothalamus, it changed how I helped my patients. It's not that I didn't know the hypothalamus existed. In anatomy and physiology courses, we learn about the brain, including the hypothalamus. But in practice, we tend to ignore it. Even though the hypothalamus maintains homeostasis – keeping in balance your metabolism, your temperature, your blood pressure, your respiration, your heart beat, and your hormones in balance – health care providers don't pay a lot of attention to it.

I found, especially in my middle-aged patients, that they're not just going through menopause. They're also having hypothyroid problems. They have low adrenal function. They might have autoimmunity, chronic fatigue, fibromyalgia. They may have other issues like cancer, or they have a history of cancer in their family that must be considered. So they're coming into menopause quite complicated.

In the late 90's, when I opened my intuitive integrative health practice, I was seeing middle aged women with quite a lot of hormonal issues. They were feeling depressed and anxious, and couldn't sleep. They were struggling with their weight. They came to me with lots of medications, but wanted to do things more naturally. So I began switching them over to bioidentical hormones and recommending nutritional supplements. But ultimately, I felt like I was giving them way too much stuff. Yes, it was natural, but I was making them dependent on all the stuff, rather than trying to get their body to function again.

So I started doing some research. I was searching for a root cause, one that would tie together the multi-branched health issues my patients were experiencing. I ended up finding a study that had been conducted on fat white mice. The researchers described behaviors and conditions in these mice that were very similar to what I was seeing in my middle-aged patients. The mice acted anxious or depressed. They weren't sleeping, and they were overweight. Their thyroid levels and adrenal function were low. When the researchers sacrificed the mice, they were able to see that these mice were not producing a key hypothalamus hormone called proopiomelanocortin. Bingo. That was it. That was the connection between all these other imbalances. With this new information, I started studying the hypothalamus.

Proopiomelanocortin (POMC) is a huge 241 amino acid prohormone. POMC gets broken down into other hormones, which control your adrenals, your thyroid, your glucose metabolism, and your day-night cycles, and the rest becomes beta-endorphins. POMC is just one of many hormones your hypothalamus produces. The part of the hypothalamus that produces POMC is the same part of the hypothalamus that controls your sex hormones. And when your sex hormones become out of balance, it affects the function of your adrenals, your thyroid, your glucose metabolism, and your day-night cycles. Going through the change affects the function of POMC.

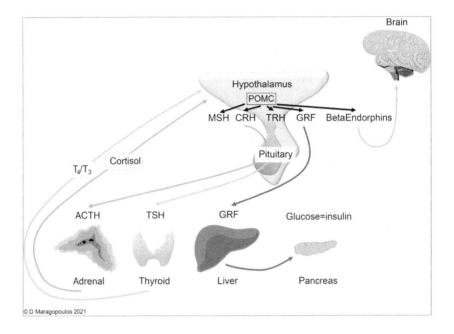

POMC controls your day-night cycles through the production of melanocyte stimulating hormone (MSH). MSH also controls the color of your hair and skin, as well as your hunger and satiety. MSH also influences your energy production. It's really an important but totally overlooked hormone. MSH is affected by your declining sex steroids, because they're controlled in the same area of the hypothalamus.

There are hormone receptors in your brain that control pretty much everything related to your body's functions. If your hormone levels drop, it's going to affect you. When estrogen drops, it affects how hungry you are, your anxiety level, your ability to remember and process information. Both estrogen and progesterone affect pain, balance, sexual behavior, and several aspects of how your brain and your body functions.

Remember, progesterone helps myelinate nerve sheaths, which ensures rapid communication in your brain. But you also have progesterone receptors throughout the brain that regulate your cognition, your ability to learn, your mood, inflammation, as well as how much energy is produced by neurons. Progesterone helps your neurons regenerate themselves, a process known as neurogenesis, which can help you recover from brain injury and aging.

Testosterone also affects your brain by helping you release dopamine. But if you have too much testosterone on board, serotonin is suppressed. There's a fine line of how much of each hormone you need in your system. So much is happening in your brain and your body during the change.

It's interesting how perimenopause is the mirror opposite of puberty. I like to take my patients back and look at their hormones over their lifespan. Starting when they were a fetus in the womb, then a child, then pubescent, then a young woman, I show the hormonal patterns they've lived throughout their lives, and where they might be declining now.

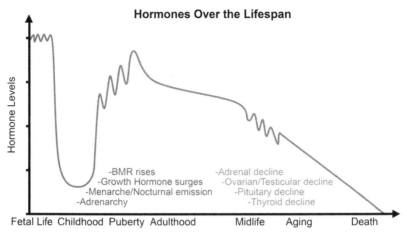

When you're a fetus in your mother's womb, your hormones are higher than they'll ever be. This is because you have to grow really quickly from a zygote to a full-term baby. And then in childhood, hormones go down to really low ambiguous levels. Little boys and little girls have similar hormone levels at that point. In pre-puberty, things start turning on. It's not your ovaries that turn on first, it's your adrenal glands. Your adrenal glands produce DHEA, which then gets converted into testosterone and estrogen. The first thing we see in puberty is hair under our armpits and pubic hair, long before periods.

Your breast buds form under the influence of the estrogen that is converted from DHEA. Then your ovaries wake up and you get your period. Menarche is the very first period. Menarche usually occurs between 11 and 15 years of age. About 18 months after you have your first period, your growth hormone surges to its peak level, and you reach your full adult height. So if you were 11 years old at menarche and not very tall, you'll reach your adult height by 13. That's what happened to my mom. She was the biggest sixth grader in her class, but then she started her period very early and didn't grow much after that, reaching an adult height of only 4'10".

After your growth hormone surges, your basal metabolic rate settles to adult levels. It's very high in puberty because you're burning energy fast to grow so quickly. That's your thyroid producing hormones to keep up with your growth spurt. By the time you graduate high school, everything levels off, and your hormones stay pretty stable throughout young adulthood.

Just as these hormones came in, that's how they go out. When you start to go through perimenopause, it's your adrenal glands that go out first. But if you're suffering from the stress of living in our modern society, your adrenal glands decline a lot sooner than they should. Adrenal insufficiency is becoming more common in women as early as their mid 20s to mid 30s.

Then, your ovaries decline and you're producing a lot less hormones. By postmenopause, you have a pituitary decline, so you're not producing as much growth hormone. You do not repair injuries as well. You bump yourself and end up with an abrasion because your skin tears so easily. Or maybe you break a bone that for an eight year old, would take maybe four weeks to heal, but now that you're 70, healing takes months.

Finally, your thyroid declines to a much lower basal metabolic rate. Average thyroid hormone production is very narrow, but you're going to see that if you were on the higher end of normal, you fall into the lower end. You may not be hypothyroid, but you're low compared to what you were as a younger person. And you can't eat as much as you used to, because you're just going to gain weight. You don't have the same energy. You're not hypothyroid yet, and you may never be in terms of blood levels, but you have lower thyroid function for you.

If your hormones fall enough, it leads to cell death because your cells cannot survive without hormones. But now that you're older, you don't metabolize hormones as efficiently or safely.

How you metabolize estrogen is of particular concern. Hormones like estrogen are growth factors. Remember, estrogen is the fertilizer, and progesterone is the gardener. Estrogen will fertilize everything in your body: your skin, your hair, your nails, your vagina, the lining of your colon, your breast cells, your uterine cells, everything. And everything will keep growing if there's not enough progesterone to tell those cells they've outlived their welcome.

Progesterone activates a gene called the p53 gene, which tells cells they need to die when they're no longer useful. For instance, when you're still reproductive and you're in the first two weeks of your menstrual cycle, you've had your period but haven't quite ovulated yet, your estrogen is at the highest. Estrogen stimulates your breast cells to potentially make milk, in case you get pregnant that month. You're not going to make milk right away, but estrogen's just priming the breasts.

Once you ovulate, you produce progesterone. Progesterone actually watches those genes. If there's no fertilization, there's no human chorionic gonadotropin (HCG) because you did not get pregnant. Because of this, the corpus luteum that produces progesterone begins to die. Progesterone then tells your breasts to settle down and stop, and your breast tissue regresses to start fresh again next cycle. If progesterone didn't control cell growth, you would continue to have stimulation month after month, and something would grow like breast cancer.

If estrogen is so stimulating, why don't more young fertile women develop more estrogen-related cancers? This can be attributed to how they metabolize their estrogen. We all make the same estrogen, and our ovaries make estradiol, a form called 17 beta-estradiol, or the most active form of estrogen. That's what your brain, skin, and eyes need to function. That's what your sex drive needs. You need estradiol, but it's very short-acting. It only lasts for a short period of time during the day. So you need to be able to convert it into the longer acting form called estrone.

Estrone is converted into fat cells. You have enzymes in your fat cells that will convert your estradiol to estrone, and you can store estrone in your fat cells. It's why women going through menopause with a little extra weight, maybe 5% heavier than their ideal weight, tend not to have as many symptoms as women who are 5% lighter than their ideal weight. That little bit of extra body fat is a buffer, and can store long-acting estrone.

Yet, estrones are not created equally. Young women tend to make what's called 2-hydroxyestrone, which is protective. If they're not converting the majority of their estradiol into safe 2-hydroxyestrone, they'll make 16-hydroxyestrone, which is inflammatory. These young women get fibrocystic breast conditions, more menstrual cramps, and menstrual migraines.

Fortunately, 16-hydroxyestrone can be converted into estriol, which is also protective. Estriol is the main pregnancy hormone. But you'll also make another type of estrone called 4-hydroxyestrone, which is is carcinogenic. When you're young, you mostly make the protective estrone and very little of the carcinogenic estrone. As you get older, you lose the enzymatic cofactors to be able to make the protective 2-hydroxyestrone, and you favor inflammatory 16-hydroxyestrone and carcinogenic 4-hydroxyestrone.

The older you are, the more overweight you are, the more alcohol you abuse, the more environmental xenoestrogens like plastics you're exposed to, the more likely it is that you're going to create inflammatory 16-hydroxyestrone and carcinogenic 4-hydroxyestrone. You can't control your age, but you can control those other things. Consuming foods rich in IC3 indoles like cruciferous vegetables, the EPA in fish oils, flax lignans and soy isoflavones can help you convert estradiol into protective 2-hydroxyestrone.

Fortunately, there are tests we can do to determine your ratios of 2-hydroxyestrone to 16-hydroxyestrone. If you were my patient, I would do a baseline estrogen metabolism test and then give you the right supplementation to actually help you convert your estrogen appropriately. So if we give you estrogen replacement therapy along with progesterone, we can try to direct your conversion.

Of course, I can't do everything for you. You're going to have to control your weight, and not abuse alcohol. You're going to have to avoid drinking out of plastic water bottles that have been overheated in the car and avoid other xenoestrogens. It's so important that you understand how your body's working, because you have control over this. Menopause is not ruling you. You have control over most everything that's happening.

Now, let's talk about what happens to progesterone. Why do you run out of progesterone first? Well, you only produce progesterone if you ovulate. Your ovaries make 95% of your progesterone, and progesterone is used by your entire body. Your adrenals can make a little bit of progesterone by adulterating pregnenolone, but adrenal progesterone becomes cortisol.

So when you're no longer ovulating or you're not ovulating regularly, you become progesterone deficient really quickly. And it begins in premenopause, really declines in perimenopause, and completely bottoms out by menopause. Without ovarian progesterone, your adrenals don't have the precursors that they need to make enough stress hormones. So you don't handle stress as well.

The normal stress response begins as a neurological response. It's like a knee-jerk reaction. For example, if I'm afraid of spiders, (I'm not by the way – I love spiders), and I saw a spider out of the corner of my eye, I would immediately startle. It's a neurological response. I don't have to think about it. There are no hormones that are produced at that point. It's my nervous system saying, *uh oh, danger!* and getting me out of the way.

As soon as that happens, my adrenals produce adrenaline to get me away from that danger. My heart rate goes up, and my blood pressure goes up so that I can escape. That's the neurological response. Except in this scenario, the spider chases me all through Ojai. I'm having to run a long way. So how am I going to get enough fuel for my muscles to get away from this thing? That's where my adrenal glands, under the influence of my hypothalamus, kick in. My hypothalamus gets triggered by the adrenaline that says, "Oh, we're being chased. We're in danger," and tells my adrenal glands to produce cortisol because I need to release the stored sugar in my muscles and liver to get away from the danger. Now I have the fuel to run away.

How did this sugar get out in the first place? Under the influence of cortisol, my pancreas releases glucagon. Glucagon triggers the release of glycogen, or stored sugar. The stored sugar floating around in my bloodstream triggers my pancreas to produce enough insulin to get the glucose into my cells – particularly the large muscles that I'm using to run away from the danger.

All of these biochemical reactions begin with a stressor that triggers your hypothalamus to tell your pituitary to produce ACTH, that tells your adrenals to produce cortisol that tells your pancreas to produce glucagon and then insulin. That is a lot of endocrine glands at work just because of one little spider.

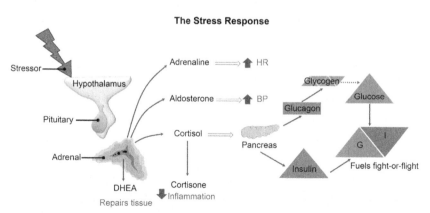

The Stress Response

© D Maragopoulos 2021

So what happens now? I've been running and running from the spider, and finally I outrun the spider. I'm exhausted, and I pulled a muscle – my hamstring. Now, how's that going to be repaired? Well, along with cortisol, my adrenals also produce DHEA. DHEA follows cortisol. DHEA helps me to metabolize protein and fat to repair those tissues.

I've talked about the stress you're not handling as well during the change. What's happening? Remember your hormones over your lifespan, and your adrenals came in first? Your adrenals start to decline first, before your ovaries, so you don't have as much adrenal support as you used to. Your DHEA levels are falling, and you're not repairing tissue as well. You may still get the adrenaline and cortisol spikes, but you don't have as much DHEA to calm down the stress response and actually repair the tissues that might've gotten hurt by the stress response.

DHEA has an anabolic effect, meaning it builds tissues. Where cortisol has a catabolic effect, it breaks down tissues. If you're constantly pumping cortisol and not enough DHEA, you're going to break down tissues like the inside of your gut and end up with a leaky gut. Then you'll have issues with certain foods. Perhaps you'll start getting eczema because your skin is reacting and cannot repair. Or your hair is falling out because you're not metabolizing protein and fat, so you can't grow healthy hair. Do you see how this is all connected? We're not just looking at your female hormones, we're looking at everything.

When you come in to see me as a patient, I want to look at everything, especially your hypothalamus. Unfortunately, we can't measure hypothalamic hormones directly, so we're going to look at other hormones that your body produces that would reflect hypothalamic function. Both your adrenals and thyroid are controlled by proopiomelanocortin, so we can look at DHEA, TSH and thyroid hormones. POMC also controls glucose function, so we'll also measure C-peptide and Hemoglobin A1c to see if you're insulin resistant. That way, we get an idea of how your hypothalamus is functioning under the stress of going through the change. Why give you more hormones than you need when we can treat the root issue?

I guarantee that if you've had multiple health issues, you definitely need hypothalamic support. If you're going through menopause, you need hypothalamic support. Supporting your hypothalamus provides the base that you need in order to use the least amount of hormone replacement therapy, as well as the least amount of estrogenic or progestational herbs. You're never going to be able to take the exact amount of hormones that your body needs on a day by day basis to replicate your hypothalamus' ability to direct your ovaries, adrenal glands, thyroid, and pancreas.

Communication between your hypothalamus and your lower endocrine glands is a very natural and organic process. No matter how good you are at following a prescription, you won't be able to match your natural rhythm of hormones. However, if your hypothalamus is supported, you're able to use the least amount of hormones, your cell receptor sites work better, your hormone metabolism is safer, and eventually you learn to listen to your body and adjust your hormones appropriately.

Your hormones affect everything, including your gastrointestinal system. If your estrogen, progesterone and testosterone levels are falling, your gut isn't functioning normally. Sex hormones improve digestion, as well as absorption of nutrients. So, it's really important we get your hypothalamus in balance because we need your gut to be as healthy as possible. If you're not digesting and absorbing properly because your gut lining is really thin, then you're not going to be able to get all the nutrition you need to actually correct your hormonal issues. That's one of the reasons that we're focusing on the big picture, not just your individual symptoms.

I want to share with you a story of one of my more complicated menopausal patients. She's a great example of what happens in your body when you actually support it from the inside out.

Layla came to me in her 50s, just as she was starting menopause, and had not been taking any kind of hormone replacement therapy. But menopause is not why she came to me. She came to me because she had chronic fatigue syndrome and was exhausted all the time. She wasn't able to walk her dogs or do any gardening, and could barely do some computer work. She spent most of her day in bed.

She also suffered from fibromyalgia, which meant that she was in pain a lot of the time. Her gut wasn't functioning normally, so she didn't digest her nutrients very well. She suffered from GERD and had chronic constipation. Because she was going through menopause, she was having trouble sleeping. She was having hot flashes, and her memory was fading with brain fog.

Layla had done a lot of research on chronic fatigue to try to figure out what was going on. She had seen many different practitioners, using lots of different natural agents, as well as functional medicine to try to fix this. But what she had not addressed was her reproductive hormones.

Her chronic fatigue had actually gotten worse as she was going through the change, and no one really looked at that. Because she had a family history of cancers, she was a little afraid of hormones. We discussed what would be safe for her, and we did a blood test to see if she was metabolizing estrogen correctly. She was actually doing a pretty good job because her diet was pretty darn clean. So we started with hypothalamus support – both Genesis Gold® and extra Sacred Seven® amino acids. The reason I recommended both is because she was one of those complicated menopause patients with other issues, particularly her autoimmune disorders, and she needed more intense hypothalamus support.

Her blood work revealed that her thyroid was low functioning. She wasn't hypothyroid yet, but it was on the low end of normal. And her adrenals were low functioning and dyscircadian. She tended to have adrenal cortisol spikes in the middle of the night and super low cortisol during the day. Rather than giving her all of those hormones, we started with hypothalamus support.

Within the first few months, she started feeling more energy, suggesting that her mitochondria had begun healing. Once we got the testing done to show that she was actually metabolizing estrogen in a pretty safe way, we went ahead and started hormone replacement therapy (HRT). It took a while to get her to feel comfortable with the prospect of HRT, even bioidenticals. We did quite a bit of work with the rest of her issues before we went that route.

With the hormone replacement therapy added to her hypothalamus support, Layla was able to get her life back. She had a lot more energy, and was able to start exercising. She was more temperature tolerant. Previously, she did not tolerate the heat at all, getting completely exhausted in the summer. By giving her bioidentical hormone replacement therapy with the hypothalamus support, she was able to tolerate the over 100 degree summer without major hot flashes and the exhaustion she would normally get.

After six months, she was able to get off the extra Sacred Seven® and continues to use Genesis Gold® to support her hypothalamus and hormone metabolism. Her chronic fatigue syndrome diminished to the point where she could play tennis.

One other interesting thing happened for Layla. She had a MTHFR genetic mutation in which she was unable to activate folic acid into its active form. Methylenetetrahydrofolate reductase, or MTHFR, is an enzyme that breaks down homocysteine, an amino acid produced when proteins are broken down. High homocysteine levels can contribute to arterial damage and blood clots in your blood vessels. Layla's baseline homocysteine levels were indicating that her

MTHFR gene was not functioning properly. After a year of supporting her hypothalamus with Genesis Gold®, Layla's homocysteine levels were normal, suggesting that she was expressing more adaptive genes.

If you support your hypothalamus, the rest of your hormone balancing is so much easier. Your hypothalamus controls everything: your weight, your temperature, your sleep cycles, your metabolism, your stress response, your heart rate, respiration and blood pressure, your salt water balance, your digestion, absorption, detoxification through your kidneys, liver and cells, your memory, focus and concentration, your moods, including depression, anxiety, panic, your reproduction, and your sex drive and sexual response.

Your hypothalamus is highly sensitive to hormonal decline. Going through the change alters the way your hypothalamus functions, which affects not just your hormones, but your overall health. It's vital to give your hypothalamus nutritional support so you do not have to use excessive amounts of hormones to overcome your hormonal imbalances, and you can live your best life.

ACTION ~ How would your life be different if you were symptom-free?

Chapter 8

The Gifts of Menopause

The change changes everything. It not only changes you physically, but emotionally, mentally, socially, and spiritually. This is the most important part of going through menopause – transforming to a more complete version of yourself.

The psychospiritual aspect of the change is probably the most significant to me. The growth that we can experience while we go through the change is so remarkable. Because our hormones are out of balance, we are forced to deal with stuff that we did not have the impetus to do before.

When you're so busy with children, your profession, and everything else going on, with hormones in fairly good balance, you're not really triggered to do your deeper soul work. But when you start going through the change, you get triggered. And if you don't deal with your soul work at this point, it keeps triggering you.

What I find is that people, whether male or female, young or old, put off the psychospiritual part of healing. The physical part of healing that I can help them with, to get everything from their hormones to their gut in balance, won't stick if they don't do the psychospiritual aspect of healing. In other words, if they don't do the soul work, they will never truly and completely heal.

I absolutely love working with menopausal women. From premenopause to postmenopause, their rollercoaster hormones trigger deeper levels of change for them. They start asking the big questions, and start making the shifts that they probably should have made 10, 20, 30 years ago. The change is the cauldron in which you can actually start simmering all of the things that need to be transformed. It's never too late because the shifts that you make now during the change will affect not just your life, but those of everyone around you.

You will be doing work that will clear up your DNA so that it's not passed on to the next generation. Perhaps you're thinking, "But wait, I already gave birth, the DNA is already in there." Yes, but believe me, your DNA resonates with other DNA. When I do my deeper work and my DNA shifts, it shifts the genetics in my children and in my grandchildren. I'm going to show you a study so you can understand this concept a little bit better. But first, let me share my own story.

My perimenopause to menopause journey lasted from age 49 to 59. A decade full of havoc but great change, probably bigger change than any other time in my life. While I had another huge decade of change between my late teens and early 20's, this was even bigger. I lost six loved ones, including my mother, which was tremendous. When a woman loses her mother, it actually shifts who she is in the circle of life, in her particular universe, and I'm going to share a little bit about that.

I had major shifts in my medical practice and my health care business. Then, my husband retired at the same time. When your partner retires, it changes the energy of your home and your relationship. Both of my children graduated from college during that period of time, both got married, one got divorced. I thought I had put a lid on the codependency and addiction that lay deep in my maternal grandfather's DNA, yet it came boiling over just as I entered perimenopause. In the midst of this, a grandbaby was born, and everything shifted. It was the most psychospiritual growth I have ever experienced in any time of my life, and I felt completely transformed from it. The change not only changed me physically, but it changed me emotionally and mentally.

Menopause is not just a physical shift. Most women are very concerned about what's happening to them physically. They want their hot flashes to go away, they want to sleep through the night, they want to get their libido back, they want to be able to orgasm again, and they want to lose weight. While these are physical changes, there are often deeply buried psychospiritual hooks that are keeping things out of balance. Fortunately, menopause is a time where everything shifts simultaneously because hormones affect every layer of your healing.

Hormones affect you physically, mentally, emotionally, and spiritually. And when I say spiritually, I'm talking about vibration. Hormones have their own vibration, and they affect what's happening within your body, as well as those around you. Hormones affect what's happening in your environment, not just the people. Your hormones affect your animals, your plants, the weather, everything. I know that sounds crazy. How can you possibly be the one to affect everything? Yet, studies show that hormones have a vibration that actually shifts the energy of things and the people around them.

You have hormonal receptors everywhere in your body. Your hypothalamus directs all your hormones and is the gatekeeper of your intelligence, your emotions, and your subconscious. Your hypothalamus also directs your genetic material. Your DNA is the holder of light vibration. DNA has a physical aspect to it, as it is nucleic acids that are hooked together. But DNA also dances, moves, shifts, and changes with vibration.

There was a study that was done on soldiers quite a few years ago that proved this dance of DNA. The researchers scraped the inside of the soldiers' cheeks to obtain genetic material. They took the soldiers' DNA into another room. They hooked the soldiers up to machines that would detect electromagnetic frequencies – measuring patterns of their hearts, brains, and muscles. Then, they had the soldiers watch movies that would induce different emotions.

They categorized the emotions as either falling in the category of fear or love. I believe emotions are on a spectrum. So everything that's loving – like gratitude, compassion, joy, and delight is on the love side. And everything that's fearful – like anger, frustration, rage, and fear is on the fear side.

The researchers observed the soldiers and their DNA, which was being measured vibrationally. When the movies were loving, sweet, and kind, the soldiers' biometrics were all in this beautiful balance, showing gentle and coherent wave formations. And their DNA was moving in the exact beautiful wave formation. When they showed the soldier something that frightened them, their biometrics showed this erratic, jagged change in the wave pattern. And the vibration of the soldiers' DNA showed the same incoherent wave pattern.

Now, this is interesting. The researchers took the DNA farther away from the soldiers. They were originally in another room, so they took their DNA 100 yards away, then a mile away, then across the country. No matter how far the DNA was away from the soldiers, if the soldiers were reacting, so was their DNA. This was a great discovery. It means that your emotions and how you respond to the world affects your genetics, as far as your DNA might go. Meaning, my DNA is in my daughter, and it's also in my granddaughter. If I'm feeling an incredible amount of fear, my daughter will perceive it as well, and so will my granddaughter.

I have been with my grandbaby, with mommy and daddy nowhere in sight, and she starts reacting. I'm talking about an infant who can't even tell you what's going on, just crying like she has been hurt, and then my daughter calls me and tells me some horrible thing that just happened to her. She's not even near the child, yet they're connected. We're all connected, and it's through this light vibration.

So what does the dance of your DNA have to do with the change? You have the unique opportunity to correct the wrongs in your DNA. I told you we were dealing with issues of addiction in the family. My grandfather was an alcoholic, though I didn't know him as one. But I grew up with a mother who was the adult child of an alcoholic, so all of the negative aspects of this– her low self-esteem, her food addiction issues– filtered down onto my sisters and me. I ended up with an eating disorder, along with two of my other sisters. It just kept filtering down through the generations.

When my daughter was five months pregnant with my granddaughter, I had a dream. The baby came to me, exactly as she is now, dark hair, blue eyes, fair skin, about four years old, and explained how she's coming to heal our lineage. I believe in dreams, I believe in vibration, and I believe if you don't do the healing work at the energetic level, then you're not going to heal at the physical level.

So how do you even begin the deeper work of the change?

If you're being bombarded by hormonal shifts and changes, you're hot flashing all the time and haven't been able to sleep because your bones are aching, you're having trouble focusing and you're moody, how can you possibly do this deeper soul work? This is where supporting your hypothalamus comes in. If you're able and willing to do that work and you support your hypothalamus, you're going to find that besides optimizing your hormones, brain, immune system, and gut, you're going to start shifting organically.

One of the reasons I created Genesis Gold® was to support us through these transitions. My intention was for this formula to help us heal – physically, mentally, and spiritually. I believed that by getting our hormones in balance and supporting our hypothalamus so that we are in homeostasis, our immune systems would function optimally, our brains and nervous systems would function optimally, our guts would function optimally, everything physical could function optimally. By supporting our hypothalamus, our mental and emotional health would improve so we could maintain those physical improvements.By supporting our hypothalamus, our DNA would actually be able to support these shifts throughout our lives.

I believe that by supporting our hypothalamus, our DNA is capable of supporting those shifts at a physical level. With this support, we could express health and well being, including aging gracefully.I personally feel that if I had not been taking Genesis Gold® from premenopause through menopause, I would not have managed the change nearly as well.

I choose to support my hypothalamus because, first, I desire optimal health. Second, because I desire to age gracefully. Yet, the main reason is because I want to be able to share my wisdom with the rest of the world. So I've got to keep everything functioning.

One of the transformational things that happens when you support your hypothalamus with Genesis Gold® during the change is the help you receive in interpreting messages from your body. Perhaps you're thinking, "My body has messages?" Of course it does!

If you were pregnant and you had cravings, those were messages. Those were messages that the baby was sending to you to tell you that you needed to eat certain nutrients for that baby's well-being. You've had messages from your body your entire life, though you may or may not pay attention to them. People who don't pay attention to the messages from their body end up getting diseases. Disease is your body yelling at you, because you didn't pay attention to its whispers.

What is your body trying to tell you?

Let's explore some of the messages that your body might be speaking to you right now during the change. These body messages are in a rainbow order, as they're associated with our chakras. Remember those seven power points within our bodies, from our root gonads all the way up to our crown pineal gland?

Our soul speaks through our body as messages, and these messages come in layers. There's seven layers of them. People consult with me and say, "Listen, I thought I got these lessons. Why do I keep reliving them?" It's because you need to understand them at higher levels.

I actually wrote this out as a document, *The Seven Layers of Soul Lessons*, and happened to have a copy of it in my guest bathroom. One day, my brother-in-law, who I wouldn't call a particularly soulful person, read it, came out of the bathroom and said, "Oh my gosh, no wonder I'm living the same issues over and over and over again. I can't seem to get through my third chakra." I was pleasantly surprised that it resonated with him. There are layers to these messages, these soul lessons. And you may relive something more than once.

I'll give you a very small example, and then I will go into each one of these rainbow colored chakras and give you an example for each of the body parts. Of course, we have many body parts with different messages, but you'll get the gist of what I'm talking about.

I thought I had dealt with my eating disorder before I created Genesis Gold®. I had gone to psychotherapy, I had been hypnotized, a psychiatrist put me on an antidepressant which didn't work, I had done all kinds of therapy. Then, I started taking the beta formula of Genesis Gold®. At that point in my life, I would say that I was on the wagon, meaning I was not indulging in my eating disorder.

Over 25 years, my eating disorder had morphed from anorexia to bulimia to an exercise obsession spotted with bulimia. I started supporting my hypothalamus, and after a few weeks, suddenly all of the donut shops in my hometown were calling out to me. I could smell donuts everywhere. I didn't even know these donut shops existed. Donuts were my bulimic drug of choice when I was in college. At the same time, I was working with quite a few different energy healers who were part of my research group, along with some of my regular patients. One of the healers said she had a similar incident where she was craving hash.

Now, I thought she was talking about corned beef hash. She wasn't. She was talking about the drug – hashish – that is a concentrated form of marijuana. She had not done anything like this for 30 years, yet she was craving it. By supporting our hypothalamus, our subconscious was talking to us. Apparently, neither of us had done the deeper work to resolve our addictions. We needed to dive deeper. My patients and customers who start taking Genesis Gold® say they start reliving old issues.

Let's say you're living in a codependent relationship with a spouse, a parent, or adult child. Now that you're going through the change, and you're taking Genesis Gold®, you're very aware of what's really going on. You're no longer willing to live in this kind of parasitic relationship where so much energy is drained from you. You desire to live in symbiosis, where there's a sharing of energy in your relationships.

This brings us to a caveat. If you choose to support your hypothalamus, be aware that you will be diving deeper into your soul work. The best part is that you'll finally get through this stuff that you've not dealt with yet. You'll finally clear the closets of your subconscious that you've not yet cleaned out.

This work is not easy, but it's necessary to live your best life. And you're not alone. Many women like you have chosen transformation with spectacular results. Let me share with you some brief stories about these soul lessons.

Whenever your body's talking to you, you can begin by asking, "What is this trying to teach me? What have I learned? Is there a gift or an opportunity here?"

So let's proceed one layer at a time – from red root gonads to the purple crown chakra.

The red root survival chakra where your ovaries lie is enlivened with sexual and creative energy. Almost 20 years ago, I had a patient who was going through the change, and her body seemed to be breaking apart. She was a very successful businesswoman, the CEO of her company, but since beginning menopause, she was in so much pain. She was having major issues with arthritis in her hips, and was barely able to move, so it was really affecting her life. She also described no libido, and no real motivation to do anything.

I'm not just a hormone expert, but also a family nurse practitioner, so I recommended intense physical therapy and supplementation to heal her inflammation so she could move forward on her healing journey. Yes, she got hormones as well, and started taking Genesis Gold®. Within two months, she suddenly decided that being a CEO was not what she should be doing with her life anymore. So she quit and indulged in a buried desire. She became an artist. And using her business connections, began selling her art. Her menopause paintings spoke to women searching for something more. She's never been happier.

That healing occurred for her because she was going through this menopause shift. Her ovaries were giving up and her energy was failing. And when she started supporting her hypothalamus with Genesis Gold®, she realized that her bliss was no longer working in the business. She wanted to do something she'd never done before. And she birthed, literally birthed, a new profession as an artist.

Now, onto the next chakra. What message might your belly chakra have for you, and how might that manifest? Bright orange, representing your pancreas, I call it the "sweetness of life" chakra.

This is your tendency to either accept the sweetness that's in life, or to reject it. Physically, in your body, it's job is to allow glucose into your cells, or to become insulin resistant. I find that my insulin resistant patients tend to have trouble living in gratitude for what's wonderful around them. The glass is half empty for them, rather than half full. So changing that mindset, that perspective, and supporting their hypothalamus makes them realize that maybe there is more to appreciate out there. It doesn't mean they're not doing the physical work, like changing their diet and exercising. It's when they are finally able to appreciate the sweetness in their life that everything shifts for them and their insulin resistance resolves.

It's a multi-layered piece of work. The physical work – following an insulin resistance diet, exercising, supporting their hypothalamus, getting their hormones in balance – and the psychospiritual work. Insulin resistance is a huge issue for women in menopause. It's another piece, another layer of healing that you may need to go through in order to be physically, emotionally, and spiritually healthy.

Next is your solar plexus chakra, the yellow one where your adrenals lie, which is also the fight-or-flight command center. This chakra is where will and emotion balance out, where you tend to react to things either fearfully or with acceptance. It's why we see anxiety with adrenal disorders. I like to help my patients understand their neuroendocrine personality by comparing them to their pets. People who are super anxious seem to have chihuahua personalities. Rather than a Labrador Retriever that's just happy-go-lucky, they're like a little chihuahua shaking in fear and barking at everything.

That kind of a nervous system creates an adrenal issue where you're constantly producing lots of adrenaline and cortisol, so you eventually wear your adrenals out. You tend to be very anxious and you make fear-based decisions. When you start supporting your hypothalamus, it starts shifting the way you react. By blunting that extreme adrenaline effect and bringing cortisol surges down, you start to mellow out. Then you get a deeper awareness of why you're reacting this way. Does that particular thing that's happening to you right now really require that level of reaction? You start asking deeper questions, and that's where the healing begins.

Again, we're still supporting your hypothalamus. If you have adrenal dysfunction and you're going through menopause, you're also getting hormone replacement therapy. Maybe you need DHEA as well. Maybe you need to be watching your diet because you have a little insulin resistance on top of this. Maybe you're reacting to certain foods. You become motivated to learn to meditate and calm down, because you're getting the deeper messages. You start to react differently to life. You learn to stop knee-jerk reactions. You begin to realize, "Oh my gosh, this is a fear-based reaction." And you start reacting in a more accepting way, which calms your body down, and calms everything around you down as well.

Now, let's move on to the heart chakra. This chakra is green, although I believe there's a pink rose quartz center in this forest green energy center. The heart chakra represents love. Green is love for everything else, and pink is self-compassion, or loving yourself.

One of the best examples of the message of the heart chakra is a perimenopausal patient. At only 48 years old, Melanie started showing signs of angina, meaning she wasn't getting enough oxygen to her heart.

When she called me with some of these signs, I immediately ordered a coronary scan. Melanie had 95% blockage in one coronary artery – the widowmaker. If it gets completely blocked, you'll have a massive heart attack and die. Melanie was really, really good at taking care of everyone else, but she was really bad at taking care of herself.

What was very interesting was that Melanie was in the second career of her life – she went from being a cosmetologist to becoming a flight attendant. Yet, she didn't get the message of this near heart attack. No, she had to get a stent placed. And only then did she start taking care of Melanie. She started supporting herself with Genesis Gold®, and began realizing there was a deeper message. Her realization occurred during a flight while she was instructing passengers before take off.

She pulled down the oxygen mask and said, "If you're sitting with someone dependent, like a child or an older person, make sure you put your oxygen mask on before you assist them." And finally, she got it. She had not been putting her oxygen mask on first before assisting others, and she almost lost her life because of that. Her story shifted, as did her health, all because of this realization.

Now we're at the fifth layer: your thyroid, or the blue throat chakra. This is about truth. Are you expressing your truth?

My patient Vicki was in a profession where she helped to train other people in public speaking, but she was really not very good at it herself. As a result, she remained in the background, helping the other speakers and not really presenting herself. Vicki also had hypothyroidism that was diagnosed in her premenopausal days and got much worse through perimenopause. As we were balancing out her hormones and her thyroid and giving her hypothalamus support, she started realizing that she wasn't speaking her truth.

She started doing that deeper level of work where she was expressing more of her truth, sharing more of her stories, what was going on for her, what she had learned in life. And she became a fantastic speaker.

What a huge difference it makes in your health and your life if you are able to understand what your body is telling you.

Now, let's go a little higher. Remember, there are seven chakras representing seven endocrine glands: red, orange, yellow, green, blue, indigo, purple. The sixth chakra is indigo, your third eye, representing your pituitary gland. This is where you gain insight. When you're going through menopause, one of the huge issues is that your pituitary hormones, FSH and LH, are crazy high. Your pituitary is screaming at your ovaries to produce more hormones. So maybe you start to get back into balance by taking bioidentical hormones, like my patient Georgia.

Georgia started to feel a little bit more in balance with BHRT, but once she began supporting her hypothalamus, she had a profound insight. She realized she'd spent her life living up to somebody else's expectations. She was fighting a little bit of weight gain in menopause, was feeling anxious, and definitely having hot flashes and insomnia. While all of that was clearing up, she woke up one day realizing that she always kept herself thin for other people – her husband, her father, her family. And at that point, her subconscious was telling her, *What about you? You need to do it for you.*

So she said, "To heck with everyone else! I'm going to do what I want. I'm going to exercise the way I want, and I'm going to eat the way I want. If this is what my body wants to do in menopause, fine." As soon as she accepted where she was at and started focusing on herself instead of living other people's expectations, the weight came off. She wasn't fighting it anymore. Supporting your hypothalamus can help you have deeper subconscious insight, and things become so much more clear.

Now we move onto the violet crown chakra, where your pineal gland produces melatonin. I believe that the message here is your connection to the Divine. How open are you to receiving information from spirit? I'm going to share my own story here. For me, this layer had to do with my connection to the sacred feminine. In my premenopause years, I really didn't feel very feminine. Now, I know now that I look feminine, and I act feminine. But at the time, in my early 40's, I didn't feel very feminine. And part of the reason is that my profession in medicine is very patriarchal, very male-driven.

I had to always prove myself with the science and the research and the case studies, and not tell any of my colleagues that a lot of what I did as a healer was intuitive. I always had the science to prove it, but it was my intuition that guided me to look in the right direction, to do the proper exam, to order particular diagnostic tests, and to be able to diagnose what I perceived in my patients. Sometimes, I would dream about patients before I ever met them and knew what was going on with them. I've always been open to divine communication, but spent the first half of my career hiding my innate knowing from the world.

I see intuition as a feminine quality. Not that men can't be open and intuitive, but women tend to be a lot more intuitive. I was denying the fullness of my gift until I started supporting my hypothalamus. By my late 30's, I was so hormonally out of balance that I needed bioidentical hormone replacement therapy. I had hypothalamic amenorrhea, meaning no periods, due to my obsessive exercise and eating disorder. I stopped all exogenous hormones when I started taking Genesis Gold®, and within two months, I started having periods on my own.

I had not had my own natural period since I was eighteen. Twenty years later, I was experiencing regular periods all the way through until menopause at 58. Having naturally balanced hormones woke something up in me: my connection to my own sacred feminine.

You may think the feminine connection is in your root chakra, but I believe it's in our crown, where we're open to everything else that's around us, as well as all those other vibrations and everyone else's emotions. We may have all our creative juices in our root chakra, but it starts with receiving information up in the crown, and then bringing it down throughout your body and then gestating, just like pregnancy.

The best ideas that actually go from conception all the way to being birthed into the world gestate for a little while. I believe that's how we work as females, as we allow those ideas to blossom and grow within us. In opening up to my sacred feminine potential, I wrote my first book, *LoveDance®: Awakening the Divine Daughter*. Writing *LoveDance®* helped me move from dry scientific jargon to rich storytelling. Sharing my stories eventually led to my second book, *Hormones in Harmony®*, which opened doorways to allow me to help so many other hormonally challenged people.

All this creative birthing began because my hormones were out of balance in premenopause. I spent years doing the soul work to really connect and be able to share with you openly how to heal yourself – body, mind, and soul.

While I have lots of research for you about how this is all connected, if you come and see me as a patient, it's not just the science that's guiding my assessment, diagnosis, or therapeutic recommendations. It's my intuition. And after 20+ years of treating the hormonally challenged, it's become very clear to me that there isn't a vat of hormones big enough to dip you in to correct all of your health problems, if we don't deal with your psychospiritual issues as well. That is going to take some time and some awareness on your part.

Shift Your Menopause Mindset

When you support your hypothalamus, it helps shift your menopause mindset from surviving to thriving.

Most of us spend our time surviving life, surviving the transitions we go through, the accidents, the mistakes, and the traumas. Yet some people thrive. Yes, they absolutely go through similar trauma, but are able to shift their perspective as they become aware of the gifts gained through their experiences and begin to thrive. Mindset shifts are transformative.

In 2017, I decided that I would teach a group of patients and customers everything I knew about hormones, from the gonads to pineal gland.. Before we started, I surveyed each participant by asking them what their main healing goal was, and what did they think kept them from reaching it? The majority said that what kept them from reaching their health goals was that they were getting in their own way, or there was something they didn't know enough about

So I shifted the program from just learning modules, and added mindset trainings. I did not prepare anything, but presented the modules and trainings as the program progressed, so I could serve the group organically. I created a support group so we could discuss what was getting in their way, and provide accountability for them. These are the same mindset shifts that we need to go through during menopause.

First is letting go of your sense of unworthiness. Many of the women I've worked with have this sense of unworthiness that presents a huge barrier to full healing. How does unworthiness manifest? Well, we do everything for everyone else and we put ourselves last, some call it martyrdom. That mindset needs to shift.

I am not saying that becoming a mindful, conscious menopausal woman doesn't mean that I don't serve and take care of those that I love, and those that are dependent on me. But it does mean I'm putting my oxygen mask on first. I'm taking care of myself physically, emotionally, mentally, and spiritually, so I can be there for them, and that includes my patients and my customers. I'm modeling how to be healthy. It's just not enough to eat well. It's just not enough to be active or to get enough sleep. It's not even enough to take Genesis Gold® to support the hypothalamus.

I have to do the soul work if this healing is going to last, if it's going to be real, and if I'm going to manifest optimal health. And so do you.

Heal your Relationships

Supporting your hypothalamus helps you heal your relationships. Women going through the change will often notice that something's up in their relationships. After 10, 20, 30 years of partnership or marriage, now their spouse is just different. Or are they themselves different?

Everybody changes. While women tend to change a little more easily than men, men's hormones follow women's hormones. When a man and woman have been partnered for a long time, their hormones follow a similar pattern. It's not unusual to see changes in a male partner after your own change, and you may even have insights before they do. I think it's a little harder to do the soul work as a male than it is as a female, because our hormones allow us to be more intuitive and open. Women get the gist of what's going on a little more easily, but it is certainly worth it to do your soul work to model for your partner, and hopefully they'll do theirs as well.

That's what I have found in my own partner. My husband and I have been together since we were 16 and 17 years of age, married just after college graduation. In over four decades, there has been a lot of soul growth. And almost always, I am the one to initiate his soul growth. I think that happens in the majority of my female patients. They will say that their male partners, husbands, or lovers don't do their soul work until they do theirs. That's just human nature. Nobody wants to change, but when things are changing around you, you've got to make a shift, or you're going to be left behind.

If you heal within yourself, you start to heal your relationships. You start really hearing what your partner is saying to you, and you start reading their messages even better. You start knowing more about how you need to show up in the relationship, because you're speaking your truth and telling your partner what you need in the relationship.

Women going through the change will complain that their libido is low, their vagina is dry, and sex is uncomfortable. Yet, once their hormones are balanced and their hypothalamus is optimized, they notice that their sex life shifts in a really amazing way. They experience better sex than they've ever had before. Everything is deeper in terms of their spiritual connections.

There are so many gifts of menopause sprouting from your seeds of intention to heal yourself – physically, emotionally, spiritually.

The change helps empower you to heal all your relationships. For example, your children are growing up and going through their own soul journeys. And as you do your work, it helps them to do theirs.

Let's say you were a helicopter parent before and hovered over your kids. You now realize that it's not helping them, and you start to pull back a little bit and do your own work. Perhaps they notice that you're getting better, and that they need to do some of their work. Even adult children may not do as deep of soul work as you're doing, because they're younger and they're dealing with different aspects. But because you're doing your work, they'll be at a whole different level than you were at their age.

Instead of focusing on their troubles, you focus on your own. You become more of a mentor to them instead of worrying about them all the time. And as you do your work, as you heal your soul, as you heal yourself hormonally, and as you come into balance, you can communicate with your children, no matter where they are in the world – and you don't need a cellphone!

You feel them. Vibrationally, things shift. It's a huge insight for you when that happens. As you're doing your work, you're seeing it mirrored in your relationships, no matter how far away your loved ones are.

Your relationship with your parents is going to shift. They're getting older, as are you. Their age is getting to the point where they may become dependent on you. So there's a shift in the relationship. You may be wedged in the sandwich generation between teenagers or college kids at home, and your dependent parents. I experienced this myself. The journey I took with my mother, from diagnosing her cancer to holding her in my arms when she died was an amazingly deep soul transformation for both of us.

At this time, my father is still very dependent, and while there's not a deep soul journeying there for him, our relationship has shifted. There's a lot more appreciation, especially on his part. I believe it's because I have shifted. He's noticed, and has said, "You're different." Which is really pretty amazing, because he's not very perceptive.

I really feel that the shift that we need to make is within ourselves. And it will shift some of these old relationship issues. Your parents may not change, they may still play the games that they've always played. But if you shift, it forces them to treat you differently and react to you differently.

This is the way the world works. Your friends are going to change around you. You may lose friends who were part of your earlier journey and don't appreciate where you're going now, and you'll gain friends who truly support where you are now. And that's a beautiful thing. Perhaps friends that fell away have now come back, and they're taking that same journey with you. Even your coworkers and workplace changes. When you heal your relationship with your work and with the people you work with, it's going to shift completely.

By the time you fully transition through the change, you're vibrating at a whole different level. When your hormones are out of balance, and you're feeling wacky and crazy, it seems like everyone around you acts wacky and crazy too. It's like being under the influence of the full moon all the time. As you become more in balance, especially if you're in a leadership position in your workplace, they become more in balance. As you change, your relationship with the earth, with the land, with the plants, with the animals shifts. You'll notice your garden, your trees, and the plants on your property start to shift and change.

There are studies that show that your health affects plants. Most of the studies are on plants living indoors with you, but your health affects outside plants, too. You have relationships with everything around you, and if you are vibrating with wholeness, health, and hormonal harmony, everything around you is at its best. And if it's not, it dies away and makes room for something new.

Recognize and Receive the Gifts of Menopause

Lastly, when you support your hypothalamus as you're going through the shift, it helps you to recognize and receive the gifts in menopause. Yes, there are gifts. I know it doesn't seem like it when you're having hot flashes, when you're struggling with your weight, or when you have brain fog. One of the gifts in menopause is that your dreams become more prolific, more vivid, more predictive, and you become a more lucid dreamer.

This happens to the majority of my patients whether they're menopausal or not, if they start taking Genesis Gold®. It might not happen right away; sometimes it takes a few months. All the physical stuff has to get healed first before they shift subconsciously. When it does happen, it's profound.

On Halloween night 2014, I had a dream. In this dream, I went to the cave of the dead. My Aunt Marie, who died in the early 80's, met me at the portal and brought me to my Nana's kitchen in South Philly exactly as I remembered it – pink linoleum, pink formica table on metal legs. The air was scented with the aromas of coffee and garlic. We sat at the table enjoying coffee and biscotti. Nana then told me what it's like on the other side. She said how we live our lives here on earth affects what's happening in heaven.

Nana explained to me so much about death and existence in spiritual form, that I've been comforted ever since. She hugged me, then took a scarf that she had over her shoulders and placed it over mine. Nana kissed my forehead and said, "This matriarchal mantle is yours now."

I was surprised. My mother was still alive at that point. "Nana, what about Mommy?" And she said, "It's your turn to become the matriarch of this family." Then I woke up.

Two months later, I diagnosed my mother with terminal cancer, and she was gone by July 2015. I had to become the matriarch and lead my family – my own nuclear family as well as my extended family. Midwifing my mother through death was one of the most profound and difficult journeys of my life, yet I was prepared because of that dream.

You will experience an increased sense of intuition. Intuition is different from instinct. Instinct is gut-based, more reactive. Intuition is within your body and your mind – a knowing about things, often without reason. You've probably experienced intuition since you were a teenager. You may or may not pay attention to it, but if you do pay attention to it, it will serve you. Your intuition becomes incredibly profound in menopause, influencing far more than your personal life.

I learned a long time ago not to ignore my intuition. I had been an intuitive child from the womb. I had a relationship with my Nana who was very intuitive, and considered a "strega" in South Philly. While strega means "witch" in Italian, these women were considered medicine women in their villages. That's what my maternal grandmother was – an uneducated, highly intuitive healer. So I was brought up with this acceptance of feelings, dreams, intuition. Yet, when I was 18 years old, one very significant time, I did not pay attention to my intuition.

One day, I was studying in the amphitheater, waiting for my boyfriend (he eventually became my husband) to pick me up from school. I was wearing heels and decided to take an elevator up to the parking lot. There was a young man also waiting for the elevator.

My intuition warned me not to get on that elevator, but my head told me, "Don't be silly." I got on the elevator and that young man assaulted me. Now, it wasn't a long elevator ride. When we reached the next floor, I was able to push him off and run away. My boyfriend saw my condition and tried to chase him down. Thankfully, he did not catch my assailant because all I could imagine was my boyfriend going to jail for beating him up. None of that happened, but I learned something at eighteen: pay attention to your intuition. I never ignored my intuition again.

Your intuition is there to serve you. Intuitive knowings and visions would come and go when I was a younger woman. Now that I'm menopausal, it's all the time. It's constant information about what needs to be done. I try to follow it as much as possible. Sometimes, it's more information than I can process.

This is one of the gifts of menopause, that you become increasingly more intuitive. You're old and wise enough and have learned enough to not ignore it. Now that you're menopausal, your wisdom has been earned. You've lived your stories.

Early in perimenopause, I attended a Grandmothers' Council where thirteen indigenous grandmothers came to my hometown in Ojai. I got to listen to these amazing women share their crone wisdom. One of the stories was from a black shaman – a priestess of the gnostic gospels, which revere Mary Magdalen as a Sophia, or wise woman. I was very interested in that particular philosophy because of my book, *LoveDance*®.

She said that when she was a younger woman, she would try to share her stories to teach other people. But all her aunties, the older women in her life, would say, "You're too young to share your stories. You haven't fully lived them." It wasn't until she became menopausal in her 50's that she finally got it. Only then had she lived long enough to understand the lessons of her stories in order for her to share them, and then be received by the younger generation.

And that's what I have found. I'm highly educated and a professional speaker, so I've had lots of opportunities to share my wisdom. Yet in my youth, I was rather evangelical about my sharing, and was just really sure that my way was the right way. Since becoming menopausal, there's no longer an evangelical molecule in my body. It's your way, it's your timing. I offer you a sip from my fountain of wisdom. If you take it, great, if you don't, that's okay too.

There's a transformation regarding your well-lived wisdom. The sharing that you will experience is one of the gifts of going through the change. What you share with others helps them on their healing journeys. By the time you're postmenopausal, you become embodied wisdom. You realize that you have a lot to share, and you're fine with sharing, and you're also fine with your audience not receiving it until they're ready.

Another gift of the change that I've experienced just as I entered postmenopause is presence. We hear about this all the time – don't live in the past, don't live in the future, live in the now. That sounds all well and good, and it's a great thing to aspire to. Now, I don't know about you, but really being fully present and living in the moment, I didn't really experience as a way of being until recently.

I've had moments of presence throughout my life. I remember so clearly breastfeeding my daughter with this amazing presence. Just imagining it, I'm back in that moment. There have been many times when I've been riding my horse and I've had this sense of oneness with everything on the trail. My breath in rhythm with hers. The sunlight glistening off the leaves of trees. Birdsong becoming so much more brilliant. Moments of presence scattered throughout my life.

Since the birth of my granddaughter, I'm living in the present more and more, to the point where sometimes, I forget to do things that I need to do because I'm so present in the moment.

It's like when you're with a little child, and you need to get to where you're going. And that little child stops in the middle of the sidewalk to appreciate a roly-poly crossing the sidewalk. Now, as a younger woman, I would rush that little child, saying, "Come on, we've got to get going." As a menopausal woman, it's all about that roly-poly. That's what's most important in the moment. And you know what? Being in the moment hasn't necessarily made me late for anything. You end up showing up on time, it may not be on the "right" time by the clock, but it's the perfect time for who needs you to be present and show up at that moment.

Being present is living like a little child, and appreciating the world in the moment. There's a lot less anxiety and worry, because you're not in the past and you're not in the future. Presence will happen more and more, and it's a beautiful place to be. This is one of the most amazing gifts of the change.

It is time for you, as a woman going through the change, to open up to your potential and intuitive empowerment and thrive. There was a time when we appreciated aging, when becoming a crone was celebrated with a crowning ceremony.

You deserve a crown for living this long to be ready to share your wisdom with others.

It's time to celebrate the crowning of your change and celebrate you as a beautiful, wise, loving, compassionate woman who's thriving through menopause, and living her best life.

ACTION ~ What gifts have you noticed so far in menopause?

Part Four

Choosing Your Vehicle

Chapter 9

Hormone Replacement Therapy

In the fall of 1999, I was asked to be part of a panel of experts. A cardiologist, an endocrinologist, a gynecologist and I were asked to help answer questions from local women being recruited for the Women's Health Initiative study.

The Women's Health Initiative was researching the effect of hormone replacement therapy in menopausal women. Funded by the American Heart Association, their goal was to see if there was less heart disease in women on hormone replacement therapy. They were using pharmaceuticals: Premarin (conjugated equine estrogens) and Provera (medroxyprogesterone).

I was concerned. The panel kept using "progesterone" to describe the progestin, Provera. I reminded them that progestins are not progesterone, noting their biochemical difference. I told them that they would not find the benefits they were hoping for if they used progestin. Although many of us were prescribing bioidentical progesterone, conventional medicine continued to prescribe synthetic progestins to prevent endometrial hyperplasia.

I was also concerned because they were using oral hormones, which would increase the risk of blood clots, in addition to conjugated equine estrones, which tend to be converted into the most carcinogenic types of estrogen.

The Women's Health Initiative study was not using the best hormone replacement therapy. Six years later, they had to close the study because they were seeing an increase in heart attacks and breast cancer. Even though the numbers were small, one in 1,500 women, people got really concerned. The media jumped on it, and women stopped using hormone replacement therapy. It was really tragic.

A lot of the women were suffering from menopause symptoms. In 1999, I tried to bring it to the attention of the researchers. When you take any steroid hormone, especially estrogen by mouth, it'll affect the clotting cascade in your liver, and increase your risk of blood clots, which will increase the risk of heart attack and stroke.

In terms of breast cancer, because they were using a progestin and not real progesterone, the women were actually not getting the protection that progesterone provides against potential cancer cells anywhere in their body. There were two arms of the study. The women who used Premarin alone actually had less breast cancer than the women who used the Premarin and Provera together. The testosterone-derived progestin actually increased the risk of breast cancer.

The Women's Health Initiative study has been analyzed more carefully since 2005 when it closed. The results showed that women who were younger, between 50 and 60, had the lowest risk of heart disease, which means hormone replacement therapy helped prevent heart disease. The only women who had an increased risk of stroke or heart attack were women older than 60 who already had coronary heart disease.

In the study, they found that in the women using estrogen and progestin for the first time, breast cancer rates did not increase significantly for seven years. However, it's important to keep in mind that we can't assume statistical significance for one type of hormone replacement therapy – oral synthetic progestin and conjugated equine estrogens – and assume other types of hormone replacement therapy are going to cause the same issues. What they found in the Women's Health Initiative study does not reflect at all on bioidentical hormone replacement therapy, or even some of the other pharmaceutical hormone replacement therapy – only Premarin and Provera.

What is the difference between synthetic hormone replacement therapy (HRT) and bioidentical hormone replacement therapy (BHRT)?

Synthetic hormone replacement therapy involves hormones that are chemically created in a lab, and have a hormonal effect in the body. The issue with Provera (medroxyprogesterone) is that it is a synthetic progestin that is derived from a testosterone molecule with fewer carbons than natural progesterone. It does protect the uterus against estrogen's building effects so that you're less likely to get endometrial cancer. But it does not protect the rest of your body, like your breast tissues. However, it is important to remember that Progestin is not progesterone.

While Premarin is extracted from horses' urine, it's a waste estrogen that your liver converts to inflammatory and carcinogenic forms of estrogen. There are other estrogens that are formulated for pharmaceutical use. Some are synthesized from bacterial RNA.

Bioidentical hormones are derived from plants, usually soy and yams. Bioidentical means it looks exactly like what your ovaries would make, so your cells don't know the difference. Bioidentical hormones still have to be synthesized somewhat, which means that you can't eat a yam and get progesterone, or eat soybeans and get estrogen. The precursor molecules of those hormones in these plants can be divided in the lab into estrogen and progesterone, as well as testosterone.

HRT and BHRT are chemically different. Synthetics are patentable, man-made chemicals. Bioidenticals are not necessarily patentable, although there are a few bioidenticals in pharmaceuticals that have patented delivery systems. You have choices.

The types of bioidentical hormone replacement therapy include estrogens – estradiol, estrone, and estriol. Sometimes they're combined, and sometimes they're taken separately.

Progesterone is best micronized, meaning it's a smaller molecule so that it's absorbed better. Chemically derived testosterone is methylated, which is very toxic to your liver. Bioidentical testosterone is non-methylated.

The adrenal hormone DHEA can also be derived from plants. Using DHEA as part of your HRT is only indicated if your bloodwork shows that you need it. DHEA is much more effective in women who actually have low DHEA levels. You want to check both the adrenal reserve with unconjugated DHEA and DHEA-S, aka sulfated DHEA, which is the active form of DHEA.

Pregnenolone is also an adrenal hormone, and is a big molecule like progesterone. Again, you only need pregnenolone if it's low on your blood work. Pregnenolone tends to be very high in puberty and adolescence, and drops naturally by the time you reach your 30s.

Human growth hormone (HGH) comes as synthetic and human-derived forms, which are absolutely bioidentical. Both are injectable and require prescriptions. HGH should only be taken if indicated, and should be paired with the proper support hormones and lifestyle to be sure the benefits outweigh the risks.

If you take high doses of something you should be making, like growth hormone that your pituitary gland produces, it'll shut down your pituitary function. Insulin-like growth factor-1 (IGF1) is a mediator of HGH that can be measured in your blood to check if you need human growth hormone.

Thyroid hormone is only indicated if your blood work shows that you need it. It should only be taken if you have a high TSH, low free T4, and low free T3, otherwise you'll shut down your thyroid. This isn't necessarily a menopausal condition, as you can be hypothyroid when you're younger, but your thyroid levels can drop as you age.

Melatonin is often used in menopause. Again, taking high doses will turn off your natural pineal production of melatonin. Care must be taken in prescribing hormone replacement therapy.

In perimenopause, I refer to hormone replacement therapy as supplemental, meaning we're just giving you enough of those hormones to help with your symptoms, but not so much that we're replacing all of your needs, because you may be able to still make it.

HRT = Symptom Relief

One goal of using hormone replacement therapy is symptom relief. Another very important goal is to prevent chronic disease. Let's start with symptoms.

Research shows that menopausal women younger than the age of 60 really do benefit from hormone replacement therapy. If the benefits outweigh the risk in a particular patient, meaning that you do not have active breast cancer or ovarian cancer, you probably would benefit from hormone replacement therapy. It's particularly effective for symptoms that are due to estrogen deficiency.

Estrogen is effective in treating vasomotor symptoms. Vasomotor symptoms include hot flashes, night sweats, nausea, dizziness, palpitations, and anxiety attacks. Estrogen also relieves secondary symptoms like insomnia and fatigue, mood changes, and concentration and memory problems. Estrogen is also very beneficial for your urogenital and sexual symptoms.

If you have vaginal dryness, itching, discharge, painful intercourse, or bleeding after intercourse, topical estrogen will help. If you have urinary frequency, urgency, pain, recurrent urinary tract infections, urge incontinence (meaning you leak a little bit or urine before you get to the bathroom), or stress incontinence (meaning if you cough, sneeze, laugh or bounce, you leak a little bit), topical estrogen will be beneficial.

Estrogen deficiency also affects your bowels. Giving hormones to women improves constipation, fecal urgency, and fecal incontinence. Estrogen helps improve urogenital prolapse, whether it's your uterus, cervix, urethra, or vagina that's sagging. Prolapse can present as a bulging in your vagina or heaviness in your pelvis. Remember, estrogen stimulates collagen which holds everything up.

Estrogen improves your sexual function, including lubrication and painful intercourse, as well as reduced genital sensation. If you have coital incontinence, which means when you have intercourse you leak urine, estrogen can help. Estrogen also improves sexual libido.

Estrogen improves so many symptoms of menopause, that it definitely needs to be considered, especially if you're younger.

How does HRT affect insomnia?

Estrogen is proven to decrease your sleep latency, meaning that you're going to fall asleep easier, stay asleep, experience fewer awakenings in the middle of the night, and fewer spontaneous arousals. Estrogen helps increase total sleep time.

Progesterone has sedative and anti-anxiety effects. Progesterone stimulates the production of GABA, which is associated with nonREM sleep. GABA calms down your nervous system. Progesterone is interesting, because it acts as a respiratory stimulant. If you have insomnia that is associated with sleep apnea, particularly obstructive sleep apnea, meaning your tongue falls back and you snore and stop breathing, progesterone has a relaxing effect to help prevent this from happening.

Of course, melatonin can be used for insomnia as well.

HRT helps treat hot flashes.

Hot flashes are best treated with estrogen. Estrogen taken in any form – orally, sublingually, transdermally – works for hot flashes.

Hot flashes are really the only FDA approved indicator for using estrogen. Otherwise, estrogen is not FDA approved for anything else, which may be a problem if you want to get your hormones covered by your insurance.

Progesterone can also be effective for hot flashes because it upregulates your estrogen receptors and suppresses luteinizing hormone. Remember, high levels of luteinizing hormone will induce hot flashes. Studies have only been done on oral forms of progesterone, and it does reduce hot flashes. Oral micronized progesterone must be taken at night because it's very sedative.

If your thyroid-stimulating hormone levels are really high, you're going to have more hot flashes. That's why it's important to look at your entire endocrine panel when getting blood work, to make sure all of your hormones are in balance.

I would rather give you a little help in all the areas you need than high dose HRT trying to overcompensate for low levels of thyroid, low levels of adrenal hormone, and low levels of pineal melatonin. It is better to take a little bit of each hormone you need than lots of one hormone.

Think of HRT like making soup. Supporting your hypothalamus is the pot of water. Estrogen is the salt. But you need the other spices, otherwise it just tastes like salty water. The other hormones are the herbs and spices that create balance. That's why we need to look at all your hormones. It's not just about estrogen – it's also about all the other hormones that your body may need during the change to improve your symptoms.

HRT treats genitourinary symptoms.

While vasomotor symptoms will dissipate with time, genitourinary symptoms develop progressively over the years. You'll pass through the hot flash phase because your hypothalamus eventually gets used to the fact that you're out of estrogen, though it may take 10 years. But your vaginal and urinary issues are going to get progressively worse without hormones. Genitourinary dysfunction affects 30-50% of menopausal women, including sexual dysfunction, vaginal dryness and pain, incontinence, and frequent urinary tract infections. Usually vaginal dryness during sexual arousal is your very first symptom. A woman may say, "No, I don't feel dry." But if they're always having to use a lubricant, that's the first sign that they don't have enough estrogen.

When I'm doing a pelvic exam on a woman who tells me that she does not have any vaginal dryness whatsoever, and I see she's got tissue paper stuck to her vulva, that's a clear sign that her vagina is becoming estrogen deficient. Oftentimes, we're not paying attention to our vaginas until we're having pain. Once you have painful intercourse, chances are that it's been going on for a while.

Estrogen deficiency causes vaginal atrophy, meaning the vaginal cells are shrinking, producing less fluid, and leaving the tissue thinner, and with less tone. There's quite a bit of evidence that using estrogen to support vaginal atrophy acts as a prophylactic to prevent urinary tract infections.

Systemic hormone replacement therapy, meaning that you're taking HRT transdermally, sublingually, or orally, does not effectively treat vaginal atrophy. You need to use estrogen directly in the vagina to provide complete relief of vaginal and urinary symptoms.

Even women who are not candidates for systemic estrogen therapy, for example, women with active cancer, can still use estrogen vaginally. Less than 25% of topical estrogen is absorbed through the vagina and into the bloodstream, so it's considered safe.

Clinically, I find that if your vagina is incredibly atrophic, meaning the tissues are dry and very thin, that there's almost no absorption until your vagina gets healthy. So what I usually do is prescribe estrogen at higher levels to get your vagina healthy, and then drop it down to less and less estrogen over time to control the systemic absorption, especially if you have breast cancer.

HRT = Protection

One goal of using hormone replacement therapy is to treat menopausal symptoms. An even more important goal of using HRT is protection. When your estrogen and progesterone levels start to fall, your risk for other diseases rises.

Osteoporosis is one debilitating disease you want to prevent.

One out of three women over the age of 50 will experience an osteoporotic fracture in her lifetime. When estrogen becomes deficient, you are going to lose bone, because estrogen stops bone loss. When you add estrogen to a menopausal woman's regime, it will decrease the resorption of her old bone.

Your bones have two types of cells. The osteocytes called osteoclasts eat up old bone, which is called bone resorption. The osteocytes called osteoblasts build new bone. Osteoblastic activity forms the amino acid matrix for the bone, and then lays down all the bone minerals. Estrogen only affects the resorption side of bone growth. It does not affect the building side of it.

When you become estrogen deficient and you're losing bone faster than you can build it, you're going to have a net loss of bone. Osteopenia is the medical term for early bone loss, which can become osteoporosis. Osteopenia means you've lost a little bit of bone, osteoporosis means you've lost enough bone that now you have a fracture risk.

The Women's Health Initiative study found that estrogen reduced fractures in women 50 to 60 years of age. But to build bone, you need progesterone, testosterone, DHEA, human growth hormone, minerals, and weight bearing and resistance exercise.

Melatonin may increase the bone density in your spine, but it does not affect your hips. We don't know for sure how melatonin affects bone density. One theory is that when you go into a deeper sleep under the influence of melatonin, your human growth hormone levels work better so you're laying down more bone.

There are medications you can take for bone loss, but they have a lot of side effects. The main medications are bisphosphonates. They help reduce bone resorption like estrogen does, but they can cause gastrointestinal irritation.

There are some new osteoporosis treatments that are being developed. Monoclonal antibodies are being studied to see if they can increase bone density by building bone. We don't have bone building drugs – we only have bone-building hormones and activities.

If you really want to benefit from healthy bones, you need to take hormone replacement therapy for at least five to ten years. Once you stop taking hormone replacement therapy, you'll start losing bone again. In my patients with osteoporosis, they use hormone replacement therapy for a long time, much longer than my patients who have healthy bone density.

It is possible to rebuild your bones completely and reverse osteoporosis, but that takes full hormonal replacement therapy, meaning you take all the hormones needed for growing bones, as well as enough estrogen to stop bone loss. The short two to five year period of hormone replacement therapy, typically prescribed by most health care providers, will provide symptom relief, but will not provide long term protection against bone loss. For that, you would need to use HRT longer.

What about your heart?

Does HRT provide cardiovascular protection? When you use estrogen in postmenopause, HRT positively affects endothelial vasodilation. This means that your arteries will open up a little bit, bringing high blood pressure down, and better blood flow to your brain, heart, and all your vital organs.

Hormone replacement therapy changes your lipid profile in a good way. HRT raises HDL cholesterol and lowers LDL cholesterol, especially the small particle size, which helps decrease the risk of plaque forming in your arteries. Estrogen therapy will help reduce the risk of developing coronary heart disease by 40-50%.

That's good news, because heart attacks kill many more women than breast cancer. Although osteoporosis won't kill you directly, if you break a hip when you're 80 to 90 years old, you have an increased chance of dying from pneumonia or a blood clot. However, it's usually your heart that takes you out. Cardiovascular protection is the most important reason for using hormone replacement therapy.

The main problem is that the benefits of HRT only last a few years after stopping it. If you never use hormones, once you go through menopause, your cardiovascular profile will look like a man's within a few years. Menopausal women have the same risk factors as men, because men don't have estrogen to protect them. The Women's Health Initiative study found that in women 50 to 60 years of age, estrogen actually did prevent heart attacks, compared to women who did not use estrogen.

What about your brain?

Does hormone replacement therapy provide neurocognitive protection? Perimenopause is the critical period for estrogen and progesterone benefits on the brain, not menopause. Of course, HRT will help you in menopause, but you start losing brain function in perimenopause when your hormones are rapidly declining.

This is why I want you to develop your Menopause Action Plan as early as possible, so by the time you reach perimenopause, you actually have a viable plan for hormone replacement therapy. In perimenopause, HRT is supplemental since you're already making some hormones. When you initiate hormone replacement therapy close to menopause, it definitely provides neuroprotection, and reduces neuro-degenerative disorders, like dementia and Alzheimer's. So you definitely want to get hormone replacement therapy onboard sooner rather than later.

But what about breast cancer?

This is what scares women the most. Which women are more at risk for breast cancer and need to carefully consider HRT?

About 80% of all women who are diagnosed with breast cancer are over the age of 45. While breast cancer is not as common in younger women, it's much more aggressive. Breast cancer risk increases with age. Between the ages of 40 and 50, one in 68 women will develop breast cancer. Between 50 and 60, one in 42 women, and between 60 and 70, one in 28 women. Your risk increases if your period started before the age of 12, or if you went through menopause naturally after the age of 55. If you have a family history of breast, ovarian, colon, or prostate cancer, you may have an increased risk for breast cancer. If you're currently using birth control, you have an increased risk of breast cancer.

However, it's not uncommon for gynecologists to prescribe birth control pills as hormone replacement therapy for perimenopausal women. Birth control pills are not the best way to control symptoms, because they increase breast cancer risk. What's unfortunate is that most women are offered synthetic hormones rather than bioidentical.

Micronized progesterone does affect the mammary gland, or the breast, in a positive way. If you use estrogen with micronized progesterone, there is not an increased risk of breast cancer for up to five years during the treatment.

Unfortunately, there isn't a lot of research on bioidentical hormones, so we really need to look at your risk factors. Honestly, I give progesterone to all of my patients who are using estrogen, whether they have a uterus or not, because I'm banking on the fact that progesterone has a protective effect in the breast, as well as other parts of the body. I believe using progesterone is safer than not using it as part of HRT.

Seven out of ten breast cancers are hormone receptor positive, which is actually not a bad thing. The hormone receptor negative cancers are much harder to treat. If you do develop breast cancer while you're taking hormone replacement therapy, you probably will have hormone receptor positivity, for both estrogen and progesterone, if you're taking both. It'll be an easier breast cancer to treat than if your breast cancer does not have any receptor sites that are positive for hormones.

It's best to make sure that you're as balanced as possible. While there are studies which advise against using hormones, as well as opposing studies that show progesterone is protective in breast cancer, you really need to pay attention to your personal risk factors.

Women who have very high natural progesterone levels in postmenopause may be at increased risk for breast cancer. This may be because these women have very high adrenal function, which is increasing progesterone levels, and more importantly, cortisol levels. Stress can increase breast cancer risk. Yet studies show that postmenopausal women with very low estrogen levels and high progesterone have decreased breast cancer risk. It's one of those crazy phenomena we're trying to figure out, which is why it's important to individualize therapy for each woman, and not decide therapy based on the average research subject.

I've had breast cancer patients who've gone through treatment, yet feel like they cannot live without their hormones. The change is drastically affecting their memory, their moods, their sex life, their sleep, their weight, and their bone density. Once they're five years past breast cancer and considered breast cancer free, they may consider using hormone replacement therapy. Again, it's a very individual decision.

There's little risk in offering vaginal estrogen to a woman with breast cancer. And there are women who will choose to use systemic hormone replacement therapy because their life is so out of balance. Younger breast cancer patients who took medications that blocked their hormone production, and caused a chemical menopause, have more issues with cognitive function, sexual function, and bone loss, and are at an increased risk for heart disease.

What about testosterone?

Testosterone can be part of hormone replacement therapy for menopausal and postmenopausal women. Yet, testosterone is tricky. Women who use testosterone have an increased risk of breast cancer in postmenopause, independent of how much estrogen they've used.

That's because testosterone is a growth factor, and can be converted into estrogen. Patients come to me on only testosterone, particularly in pellets, thinking it's safer. However, testosterone alone is not safer. You need to make sure that you're getting the proper hormone replacement therapy in order to be as safe as possible against cancers that may be hormonally fed, as well as protection against diseases like cognitive dysfunction, osteoporosis, and heart disease.

What's the difference between systemic and vaginal therapy?

Systemic hormone replacement therapy means that if you take it, you are going to have hormone effects all over your body – your brain, your heart, your blood vessels, your bones, your breasts, your uterus – everywhere. Local HRT, like vaginal estrogen, is considered topical, affecting just the urogenital area.

Vaginal estrogen affects the bladder and vulva, but it's not affecting the rest of the body. Systemic estrogens are delivered orally as pills or capsules, sublingually as tablets, oils, or mists, transdermally as patches, gels, lotions, or creams, or as injections or pellets. Vaginal estrogen is usually going to be prescribed as a cream, but it can also be insertable tablets or rings. I don't find that the tablets absorb very well.

The FDA has approved estradiol in many different forms, and micronized progesterone, both orally and vaginally, although the vaginal forms are only approved for infertility. Vaginal progesterone is not used for hormone replacement therapy. It could be, but that would be considered off-label.

If you want to have a more personalized hormone replacement therapy experience, meaning more precise dosing in a delivery mechanism that works best for you, then it's best to get your bioidentical hormone replacement compounded by a trained pharmacist. BHRT can be compounded to be delivered orally, by pellets, transdermally, and sublingually (underneath the tongue), as well as vaginally.

Pros and cons of different delivery systems

Oral HRT or BHRT is the most commonly prescribed method. That's because oral pills were the first delivery system. You can pretty much take any hormone orally. But there's a big problem with oral hormones. Steroid hormones, those large hormones with a cholesterol molecule in the middle of them – estrogen, progesterone, testosterone, cortisol, DHEA, and pregnenolone – can cause blood clots when taken by mouth. Steroid hormones have to be processed by the liver. When you take them orally, they go through your liver twice and interfere with your liver's clotting cascade. If you take steroid hormones orally for months, you're going to have an increased risk of throwing blood clots.

There are some small studies showing that oral micronized progesterone is less likely to cause blood clots and may be safer. Oral hormones can be used very short term, but they're not good for replacement therapy, which is a long term prescription.

What about sublingual?

Sublingual means underneath the tongue. So how's that different from oral? By taking a hormone sublingually, you're getting the majority of the hormone directly into the bloodstream through the big blood vessel right under your tongue. There's very little oral absorption, meaning you're not swallowing it, so it's bypassing the liver. Sublingual hormones actually work a lot faster. You get the effect very quickly. You don't always sustain the effects, so it has to be dosed more frequently – at least twice a day, or sometimes more.

I like sublingual hormones. They're a great rescue measure for my patients who are very deficient. I use sublingual estradiol for women with migraines as a preventive. Taking estradiol sublingually right before or during their period works quickly to prevent, and even abort, a migraine. FDA approved estradiol tablets dissolve under the tongue and work well.

Unfortunately, it can't be prescribed that way, meaning if your prescriber writes *sublingual*, the pharmacist will say it doesn't come that way. But the tablet does dissolve. In fact, you can put that tablet into your vagina and it will dissolve. We used to do that with birth control pills in women who get very nauseated with the pill. Tablets dissolve under the tongue, but capsules do not. There's also sublingual oils and mists that compounding pharmacists make.

What about pellets?

Pellets are hormones pressed into small cylinders that are injected under the skin. Pellets are similar to birth control implants in their delivery mechanism, and are usually compounded. Hormone pellets are meant to last three to five months.

Pellets used for hormone replacement therapy are not placed in the arm, but in the fat of the buttocks. And they're usually testosterone and estrogen. There is little information available that shows that progesterone in pellet form can protect your uterus from endometrial cancer.

Twenty years ago, I had a few patients interested in trying pellets for hormone replacement therapy, so I did a little research. Pellets use bioidentical hormones, and are created in a compounding pharmacy so I could individualize the dosing. Pellets weren't good at delivering progesterone, so we still had to use progesterone in a different form, usually transdermally.

The issue I found with pellets is first, you need to have them injected every few months. Number two, we cannot control the amount of hormones you're going to absorb. Even though pellets are compounded to the prescriber's recommendation, some women's bodies suck the hormones out quickly, giving them super high levels initially, which may give them extreme side effects, but then the effects wear off. Some women barely get any hormone from the pellets, and so it lasts a long time in their system. We can't control it. So if it's not going to work for you, you're stuck with those pellets until they dissolve, which could take three to five months.

Although I'm not a big fan of pellets as a form of hormone replacement therapy, it's an easy way for providers who don't know much about how to prescribe hormone replacement therapy to send their patients' blood work to the pellet company and have the pellets compounded for that particular patient. The problem is that blood work does not always reflect your hormone needs, determined by your symptoms, your risk factors, or your history. Your pituitary FSH and LH are more reflective of how much of each hormone you need at any particular point in the change. I don't go by your blood levels of estrogen, progesterone, and testosterone to determine the dose of hormones you're going to need, because your tissue levels and what's floating around in your blood are two different things. Since the dosages cannot be adjusted for at least three months, I don't use pellets in my patients.

What about transdermal hormones?

I use more transdermal hormones in my patients than any other delivery mechanism. This is because they're easy to use. My patient can apply them herself, and isn't dependent upon me. I like to teach my patients how to use a little more or a little less according to their symptoms. Transdermal hormones are very adjustable. With guidance, you're able to use more when you need more, and less when you need less.

Unlike pellets, you're able to take a break from hormones once a month. I give all of my patients a break from estrogen, progesterone, and testosterone three days out of every calendar month. The reason I do that is because it takes 72 hours to clear your receptor sites of the hormones, so that on the fourth day, when you restart your hormones, it's fresh again. Otherwise, after about nine to ten months, you will become desensitized to hormone replacement therapy. It's not going to feel the same anymore. That's because your hypothalamus thinks you've been pregnant this whole time since you haven't taken breaks like a period to actually clear your receptor sites.

So I prescribe hormones with a 72 hour break each month. Not all women tolerate stopping their hormones for three days. It matters how much reserve hormones you have in your fat cells to carry you through the break. But taking a break does help to make the hormones feel fresh in your body so that you don't have to keep using more and more hormones to control your symptoms.

Transdermal hormones can be compounded into creams, gels, and lotions. If the cream, gel or lotion is a water or alcohol base, it is not going to deliver the hormone as effectively through the skin and into the subcutaneous tissue. A true transdermal delivers hormones all the way through the skin and into the subcutaneous fat to be absorbed into the bloodstream. Steroid hormones are best delivered in a liposomal, or fat-based, carrier.

Most compounding pharmacies are not proficient at making liposomal bases. Because of this, we get very different results with transdermal hormone replacement therapy. It's why a lot of health care providers won't prescribe BHRT, because they don't get effective results with them. They're using the wrong base.

Liposomal bases are more expensive to make, but they deliver the hormones more effectively. With alcohol bases, the hormone doses have to be much higher. You need to use a lot more cream to get adequate absorption. Studies show that these alcohol-based creams just sit in your skin, and often do not even reach your subcutaneous fat, which means they're not getting into your bloodstream.

Transdermal patches are FDA approved to deliver hormones, yet they only deliver estradiol, not bioidentical progesterone. The combo patch contains progestin, not progesterone. Some women love the convenience of patches. I found that the patch did not stick properly, and was constantly falling off, leaving a circular irritation on my skin. I personally use liposomal BHRT.

How much BHRT should you use?

I dose my patients individually, meaning every woman takes a different amount of hormones prescribed particularly for her.

Remember, there's three types of estrogen - estradiol, estriol, and estrone. I don't use estrone; I only use estradiol and estriol. This is because your body is going to convert the estradiol into estrone naturally. And I have not found a source of estrone that guarantees it's safe to use.

I would rather help you control the way you metabolize your estradiol into safe estrone by making sure you're taking the supplements, consuming the right diet, and living the lifestyle that will help you metabolize your hormones safely. I would rather not give you the carcinogenic or inflammatory type of estrone. If you mix estradiol, estriol, and estrone together, it's called Tri-est. I don't prescribe Tri-est, but I do prescribe Bi-est, which is estradiol and estriol together. I don't use the estrone aspect of it, because I can't control what you're actually getting.

Estradiol doses usually range anywhere from 0.5mg to 2.5mg daily. There are protocols using much higher dosages trying to get women into reproductive levels of estrogen. The issue with high dose HRT is that postmenopausal women do not metabolize estrogen safely, which may increase the risk for estrogen-fed cancers. I tend to use lower doses of estrogen, and then support your hypothalamus and estrogen receptors so that less is more effective.

Estriol dosage is between 2-8mg. It's almost never given by itself, and is usually given with estradiol, because you can't convert estriol back into estradiol. Estradiol can be converted eventually into estriol, but not the other way around. Estriol will not improve cardiovascular function or neurocognitive functioning.

Estriol is great for your tissues, your bladder and vagina particularly, which is why I recommend using estriol vaginally. Vaginal estriol dosage is usually 1-2mg nightly to heal atrophic vaginitis. I find that six to eight weeks of two milligrams nightly, and then cutting down to one milligram, and then maybe every other night after that works well for most women.

Progesterone is micronized for best absorption. Transdermal progesterone has to be in a liposomal base, because it will not absorb very well in a water-based gel or alcohol-based cream. The dose is usually between 25 to 200 milligrams daily. The FDA has approved 100 mg micronized progesterone capsules. The dosage can actually be lower if you have a good delivery system, or higher if you do not have a good delivery system.

Testosterone dosages are usually one to two milligrams per day. Most women do fine on one milligram per day. I've seen women dosed incredibly high with testosterone. At first, they feel great – more motivated, stronger, high libido – but high dose testosterone has all kinds of side effects.

Most women will get whiskers, sometimes acne, and may lose hair, often in the male pattern. Of even greater concern are cardiovascular issues – increased cardiac reactive protein, increased inflammation, arteriosclerosis. High dose testosterone is not great for women, so I do not recommend it. You may not even need testosterone. I do look at blood testosterone levels, and always give estrogen and progesterone first, only adding testosterone later if we're not seeing an increase in libido. I do use testosterone in women with osteoporosis, because it's great for bone building.

Where's the best place to apply transdermal hormones?

I recommend applying transdermal hormones on your upper inner thighs. That way, BHRT gets into the highly vascular brown fat for the best systemic effect. I do not recommend applying transdermal hormones to the thin skin of your inner arms or neck. The effect may be faster, but will not last as long, so you'll have to dose frequently. Do not apply hormones to abdominal fat because absorption is poor.

Of course, vaginal estriol is applied vaginally. I prefer for my patients to use their fingers to really get a good application of cream around the entire introitus, or opening of the vagina. Paying particular attention to the top of the vagina where the urethra lies can help with stress incontinence. If your vagina is atrophied, at first you'll notice how thin your tissues are. After eight weeks, you'll notice a healthy thickening and more moisture, which is a good sign. If you use an applicator, you will not get as thorough absorption and you have to use a lot more cream.

Sometimes with testosterone, I have my patients initially apply it to their clitoral area before moving to the groin. You only have estrogen receptors in your vagina, but you do have testosterone receptors around your clitoris.

What about the other hormones?

Dehydroepiandrosterone or **DHEA** is taken only if you actually need it. I base my DHEA recommendation on blood levels. As you get older, DHEA naturally falls. The norms of DHEA levels have fallen over time. What was considered the norm 25 years ago was double what's considered normal now. And that's across the age groups and in both males and females.

Our DHEA levels have definitely dropped, and I believe that's because we're under so much more stress. We actually make less DHEA because we're making less cortisol. Lab norms are just what everyone else is making, yet it's not optimal.

Optimally, I'd like to see your DHEA-S around 100. Women are super sensitive to DHEA supplementation. Some women do great with DHEA, while other women turn it into testosterone and experience whiskers, acne, and irritability. Every woman is different in how she might respond to DHEA. I recommend DHEA to be taken sublingually, or underneath the tongue, about 25 milligrams, up to 50 milligrams a day. I only have my patients take it six days a week to give their adrenals a chance to make their own DHEA.

You're not going to be on DHEA forever unless your adrenals don't kick in. If you're younger, your adrenals are more likely to kick in and produce adequate amounts of DHEA. If you're postmenopausal, your adrenals may not. DHEA, at the 25 milligram dosage taken six days a week, is usually enough for most women. Once we get their levels up, we start cutting down how many days a week they take it. So very few of my patients take DHEA for a long period of time.

Now, some women are so sensitive to DHEA even in the sublingual form, that they will convert it into testosterone and develop acne and hairiness. These are usually young premenopausal or perimenopausal women with adrenal insufficiency, not postmenopausal women. So I offer them 7-keto DHEA, which only comes orally, not sublingually, and they can only use it for a short period of time to prevent blood clots. I use this activated form of DHEA because it cannot be converted into testosterone. For most women, we want some testosterone conversion to help build muscle and bone.

Pregnenolone is another adrenal hormone that can be taken orally or sublingually. I prefer sublingual to oral. The dose is 15 to 30 milligrams for six days a week, to prevent shutting down your adrenal glands. I only recommend it if your levels are low.

Remember, your levels are naturally going to fall as you get older. All our hormones are higher when we're in puberty, but pregnenolone is particularly high. By midlife, pregnenolone levels usually range between 33 and 248 ng/dl, with the higher levels being in 18-30 year olds, and the lower levels being in 60-80 year olds. If we can keep your pregnenolone between 30 and 50 ng/dl postmenopausally, that's pretty good.

Now, let's look at human growth hormone.

Human growth hormone or HGH is kind of tricky. Real HGH is a very expensive injectable prescription medication. I only use it in my patients who are HGH deficient and have osteoporosis. I don't use it for all of my patients who have low human growth hormone. I usually get a pretty good effect by giving them amino acid precursors to make their own human growth hormone. Arginine is the main amino acid precursor, but there are quite a few co-factor amino acid precursors that work together, and can help to boost human growth hormone production.

Like all the rest of hormone replacement therapy, you need to take a break from using HGH amino acid precursors, or you will overwork your pituitary gland. So it's best to do three months on the amino acids, and then we can recheck your insulin-like growth factors or IGF-1 levels. Remember, we're not measuring human growth hormone, we're measuring IGF-1, the mediator of human growth hormone. We can't really measure your human growth hormone without putting you in the hospital and taking your blood every five minutes.

Reflecting HGH, IGF-1 is highest when you're really young. By the time you reach 35 to 39 years old, you're at 50% of what you were at 18 years of age. And by the time you're 70, you're at 25%. So there's this natural decline in human growth hormone levels as you get older.

I give my patients the amino acid precursors for three months, and then I have them take a month off so their pituitary gland can rest, and then three months on and one month off. I always check their IGF-1 within those first three months to make sure it's rising. I use it to help build bone, but it's not the only hormone. To reverse osteoporosis, you need estrogen to stop bone loss, and progesterone, testosterone, and DHEA to build bone.

So what about thyroid hormone?

Do all menopausal women get thyroid hormone? Absolutely not. You would only get this if your blood levels are low, indicating you're hypothyroid. Giving thyroid hormone to someone who's both overweight and tired, with normal TSH, T_4 and T_3 is going to stop her thyroid from producing its own hormones. You have to be really careful with overusing any hormone replacement therapy if you want your own glands to be able to make their own hormones. If your thyroid has been surgically removed, you will need thyroid replacement therapy for the rest of your life.

Thyroid hormone can be prescribed as a synthetic, a glandular, or a plant-derived bioidentical compound. It's almost always dosed orally. Unlike steroid hormones, thyroid hormone is so small it does not cause blood clots when taken orally. Thyroid hormone can also be compounded into a transdermal cream. I prefer compounded thyroid hormone because it's very precise. I can give you exactly the amount of T_3 and T_4 that your body needs in a sustained release compound so that you can take just one pill in the morning and you're good.

There are FDA approved desiccated thyroid extracts that come from the thyroid glands of either pigs, sheep, or cows. The ratio of T_4 to T_3 is always the same. Sometimes it's too much T_3 for patients, and sometimes it's too little, which is why I prefer compounding thyroid hormone.

Typical doses of T_4 are usually 15-110 micrograms, and T_3 is between 3-25 micrograms. I rarely ever need 25 micrograms of T_3 because my patients get holistic hormone replacement therapy. If my patient is low in thyroid and she's also menopausal, she's going to get estrogen and progesterone before we're even going to give her any thyroid hormone. Estrogen helps to enhance T_3 uptake so we get more bang for our buck. We want to make sure that we're paying attention to all of her hormones, not just one hormone, like thyroid.

Melatonin is also very useful as women go through menopause. Your melatonin levels drop as you age, which is why older people sleep less hours at night than younger people. Under the influence of melatonin, your immune system functions better. Melatonin helps you sleep a little bit deeper.

Melatonin doses are between 0.5 to 5 milligrams, and are either fast acting or sustained release. Fast acting means it works really quickly and you can go to sleep very soon after taking it. Sustained release melatonin is not going to kick in until later. It's better for women who are waking up in the middle of the night to use sustained release melatonin.

Although you can get higher doses of melatonin over the counter, if you use a higher dose, you may shut your pineal gland off. So I try to keep the doses a little bit lower. I prefer the sustained release to keep you asleep, in addition to using something else to put you to sleep, like progesterone..

Do you have to take hormones forever?

Using hormones past menopause is an individualized decision. European studies demonstrate that women taking hormones into their 80s have no adverse effects. I have a few patients in their 80s that still take hormones.

It's possible to continue to take hormones for many decades and not have an increased risk of cancers. Using HRT in your senior years is a very individual decision, and you need to take into account your genetics, family history, and your current and past lifestyle. Every woman is different.

I had a couple patients who would come to my office together, one in her late 70s, the other in her early 80s. Both were using hormone replacement therapy systemically, as well as vaginal estrogen, because they were both sexually active. In fact, they were single women who liked to go to bars together. They would arrive in my office to make sure that their vaginas were nice and healthy before they would go out.

It's not my decision as a health care provider; how long you want to use hormones is your decision.

Can you start hormone replacement therapy if you're postmenopausal? Absolutely. If you went through menopause and didn't use any hormones and now you have osteoporosis, an incredibly dry vagina, and you want hormones, you can absolutely start them.

We just need to make sure that you don't have active breast cancer, so we may do breast imaging to be sure that HRT will be safe for you. And even if you do have breast cancer, you can still use some vaginal estrogens. Older women may need hormone replacement therapy, and should be given the opportunity to discuss the risks and benefits with their health care provider.

Are you going to have more issues if you initiate hormone replacement therapy when you're older? Well, if you haven't had estrogen on board for 20 years, estrogen will wake up certain body parts. Because of this, you're going to be more susceptible to estrogen-related side effects like bloating, breast tenderness, and vaginal discharge.

Even if you're 80 years old and you take enough estrogen, your uterus lining can be stimulated, meaning you might bleed. Your tissues are still alive and viable, and hormones can bring them out of hibernation.

So you want to start out very low and slow when you first initiate hormones if you've been menopausal for more than 10 years. If you're well into postmenopause, we're going to gradually titrate your dose to reduce symptoms. You don't necessarily need high doses to get a good effect.

While there is always a potential that if you use hormones between the ages of 60 and 70, you may have some increased risk for breast cancer, the risk is different for every woman. So I make it an individual decision for each woman, and we do the appropriate screenings for breast cancers. We check bone density with a DEXA scan, and make sure that she's not actively losing bone with a urine cross link test. We check the rest of her hormones too.

I like to look at a woman in terms of her biological age, not her chronological age. For instance, I was born in 1961, so my chronological age in 2021 is 60. However, biologically, my biochemistry is more like 45. So am I going to take hormones longer? Probably, because I don't have the metabolism of a 60 year old. I have the metabolism of a 45 year old.

Every woman is different. Health care providers should consider each as an individual, and not assume that just because a woman falls into an age group that she's no longer a candidate for hormone replacement therapy. Of course, once you're done with HRT, you can stop. But it isn't wise to stop suddenly. Slowly come down, because it'll be a shock to your system and will feel like you're going through menopause all over again.

One way that you can use hormone replacement therapy for long periods of time, well into postmenopause, is by giving yourself hypothalamic support. If you decide you're going to support your hypothalamus with Genesis Gold®, it's going to increase your cell receptor site activity, so you can use less hormone replacement therapy. That's why the dosages I recommend for HRT are much lower than typical dosages, because the majority of my patients are supporting their hypothalamus with Genesis Gold®. They can use a lot less hormones and get the same or better results.

When you support your hypothalamus, you're improving communication between the hormones you're taking, like sex hormones – estrogen, progesterone and testosterone – and your hypothalamus and pituitary. Supporting your hypothalamus also improves communication between all your other hormones. Using Genesis Gold® helps improve adrenal function, supports growth hormone production, and even supports other pituitary hormones, like oxytocin, so you have better orgasms. It also improves your brain function, your immune function, and reduces the symptoms of menopause.

One nice benefit of supporting my hypothalamus is that instead of bumping up my hormone replacement therapy when I'm under stress, I just take extra Genesis Gold®. In more extreme cases, meaning the stress is very high, (like the seven months I took care of my dying mother), I add a little extra Sacred Seven® amino acids. Many of my patients and customers use extra hypothalamus support when they're under increased levels of stress.

Stress can induce symptoms of menopause like night sweats and brain fog, even if you're on HRT. Supporting your hypothalamus with Genesis Gold® helps diminish the effects of stress.

You have a full spectrum of choices while going through the change. HRT is one of those choices. However, there are also alternative treatments that can be used instead of, or in addition to, hormone replacement therapy.

ACTION ~ What type of bioidentical hormone replacement therapy do you need?

Sex Hormones - systemic and topical	Other Hormone Replacement Therapy
Estrogens: Estradiol, Estrone, Estriol	DHEA
Progesterone	Pregnenolone
Testosterone	Melatonin
Vaginal estrogen	Thyroid - T4/T3
	Human Growth Hormone (HGH)

© D Maragopoulos 2021

Chapter 10

Alternative Therapies

As a hormone expert, I guide the majority of my patients on the use of bioidentical hormones to help them transition through the change of life. Yet there are many alternatives to hormone replacement therapy for you to consider for your Menopause Action Plan.

As a medical detective, I research the best options for each individual patient. My patients are very open to using both traditional and alternative therapies. In my experience, bioidentical hormones work the best to handle most women's menopausal symptoms. I focus the majority of alternative therapy on very particular health concerns. In this chapter, I will present the different options available, as well as their pros and cons, so you can choose what might be useful for you.

A lot of women will read information on the internet or get information from friends and family. Many will go into a health food store and see a bottle that says "Hot flash relief," and they buy it.

I'm going to go over the research behind whether or not these alternative therapies work. I want you to understand that the majority of the supplements available are combined, yet the research only looks at individual therapies. Besides the oral therapies, I'm going to go over other non-hormonal treatments that have been studied related to menopause and symptom relief. I'm also going to share with you some special protocols I've developed for my patients. By the end of this chapter, you're going to be able to make some really informed decisions about what might be the best treatments for you.

First, the basis of the support that I offer my patients is hypothalamic. I'm going to go over hypothalamus support in detail at the end. My patients come to me with a variety of different supplements they've tried without relief, or perhaps they experienced uncomfortable side effects. It's not unusual for a woman to come in with a huge shopping bag full of supplements she's been taking for her menopausal symptoms, as well as all kinds of other issues that she's dealing with. Most of the time, she's taking far more than she needs, and a lot of the supplements she's taking contraindicate each other, contributing to her issues.

I like to clean house with my patients, and have them start fresh with hypothalamic support, but I never pull the rug out from under them right away. When they start hypothalamic support with Genesis Gold®, I always have them just use whatever they've been using for about a month before tapering down. The key to keeping your hypothalamus balanced is to introduce changes carefully – whether it's supplementation, bodywork or energy therapy.

Botanical therapies

Botanical therapies are herbs or plant extracts that have hormonal effects. The most common premenopause herbal therapy is **chasteberry**. Chasteberry has a progestational effect, meaning it acts like progesterone in your body. It comes from the Vitex tree that originates in the Mediterranean. I have one of these beautiful purple flowered trees in my medicinal herb garden.

Chasteberry got its name because it was believed to decrease sexual desire. In the Middle Ages it was used by monks to help them stay chaste. Because of its progestational effect, chasteberry is effective in premenopausal women to help control irregular periods. There are no studies that support its use for menopausal symptoms.

Chasteberry seems to be effective in reducing breast pain and other PMS symptoms, like bloating and headache in premenopause. The recommended dose is 30 to 40 milligrams of chasteberry extract per day.

Black cohosh is considered estrogenic, but while it has an estrogen-like effect, it doesn't fill the estrogen receptors. Black cohosh is a member of the buttercup family, and grows in North America. It was used by Native Americans in a variety of traditional medicines for female complaints related to menstruation and childbirth.

Black cohosh appears to act on the serotonin receptors rather than the estrogen receptors, which is why it may relieve hot flashes and improve your moods. It's difficult to conclude from all the studies that have been done on black cohosh if it's beneficial by itself or only in combination with other herbs, vitamins, and minerals, because that's usually how it's found on the market.

There are some side effects to black cohosh, including gastrointestinal upset and rash. If you take a lot, and people tend to take more than they need, thinking that if a little is good then more is better, you can develop acute hepatitis. You must be careful with your dosing. Studies show for menopausal symptoms, the dose for standardized extract of black cohosh is 20-40 mg twice daily. It's best not to take black cohosh for more than six months.

Maca is a botanical used to boost male testosterone production and female libido, but it's not necessarily androgenic. Maca is a plant which grows in the Andes. It's in the brassica family, which is the same as mustard and cruciferous vegetables. It's been used for centuries for infertility and female hormone balance in the Andes.

Researchers do systemic reviews of all the different studies that have been published on a subject to evaluate results. In systemic reviews on maca, there seems to be limited evidence of how effective maca is in treating menopausal symptoms. It does seem to reduce psychological symptoms of anxiety and depression, and may lower the measurements of sexual dysfunction due to mood imbalances. We're not really sure how maca works. The recommended dose for maca is 1,500 to 3000 milligrams a day. You can get maca in a loose powder that you can add into smoothies. There's not a lot of safety information on it, so I would definitely be careful with high doses of maca for long periods of time.

Phytoestrogens are also in this category of botanicals that have effects on your hormones. Phytoestrogen means plant estrogen, and they are mainly extracted from soy and red clover. Red clover is a lot stronger than soy. Phytoestrogens seem to have a minimal effect on menopausal symptoms, but they definitely have a positive effect on your lipid profiles and balancing your cholesterol, so they may reduce the risk of heart disease. Phytoestrogens may have some potential effects on bone growth, as well as memory and cognition. Rather than taken as a supplement, phytoestrogens in your diet can be an excellent way to increase the effect of estrogen receptor sites to help improve cholesterol, bone density, and your memory.

There are a lot of other botanicals used in menopause, including hops, dong quai, evening primrose, ginkgo, ginseng, kava root, valerian root, licorice root, motherwort, St. John's root, royal jelly and wild yam. Unfortunately, there's very little data on the efficacy and safety of these compounds for long term use during the change. Oftentimes, menopausal supplements will be combined with some of these different compounds.

When I have lab results to show that my patients really need the type of support these additional botanicals may offer, I tend to use supplements that are in combination for my patients' particular issues. They're used for a limited time, usually just a few weeks and up to a few months. I would be careful with high doses of any of these herbs over a long period of time. Because the change can last from five to fifteen years or longer, it could be a long period of time you need help with symptoms. The majority of the research done on these botanicals is only for three to six months.

Aromatherapy

I frequently get asked about using essential oils for menopause. Essential oils fall in the aromatherapy category. These scented oils are believed to increase relaxation, which may be beneficial in easing menopausal symptoms. A 12-week study using lavender as the essential oil found that aromatherapy seemed to improve menopausal women's sleep, compared to just educating them about proper sleep hygiene. There was also a 12-week study that showed that hot flash frequency was reduced by 50% with lavender aromatherapy.

Lavender probably has a relaxing effect on the brain, perhaps raising GABA and affecting serotonin, which could explain how it might reduce hot flashes. Lavender is not to be eaten, but is to be inhaled. I use lavender essential oil in the bath and spray it on pillows to help with sleep and relaxation. While there definitely needs to be more studies, aromatherapy seems to be safe.

When aromatherapy is used during massage therapy, it's more effective than massage alone to relieve menopausal symptoms. I believe most menopausal women could benefit from regular massages, and adding aromatherapy with oils can make a big difference in helping you relax. A relaxed nervous system helps calm down some of your menopausal symptoms, particularly vasomotor symptoms like hot flashes and night sweats.

Vitamins and minerals

Vitamin D is the most important vitamin for women going through the change. A pro-hormone, vitamin D helps modulate your neuro-immune-endocrine system. Vitamin D is crucial in keeping hormone receptor sites active. Keeping your vitamin D at an optimal blood level is key to hormone health. While a serum 25-hydroxy vitamin D over 30 is considered normal, for optimal health, I like my patients' levels to be at least 50.

There's clearly an inverse association with how much vitamin D is circulating in your bloodstream and the risk of death due to cardiovascular disease, cancer, and other causes. The lower your vitamin D, the higher your risk of death. The recommended dose of vitamin D supplementation is according to what your blood levels are. If your blood levels are very low, under 30, I recommend bolus dosing, about 10,000 international units every day, for a few weeks up to two months to get those levels up, and then slowly bring the vitamin D supplementation down.

Vitamin D is the sunshine vitamin. If you sunbathe for at least 15 minutes a day with 80% of your body exposed, you're going to make about 4,000 international units of vitamin D. But as we get older, our skin is not as efficient at making vitamin D, which is why vitamin D levels decline with age. Vitamin D deficiency is incredibly prominent in the population, perhaps because we spend too much time indoors, and it's difficult to get enough vitamin D from your diet. What's added into milk is a plant form of vitamin D called D2. Your body needs Vitamin D3 and cannot convert D2 into D3. You need to take vitamin D3 that is animal based, which usually comes from fatty fish skin.

You can get vitamin D3 from eating fish skin. Yet most people can't eat enough fish skin so I recommend supplementing vitamin D3 when your vitamin D levels are low. I use a triglyceride form of vitamin D3 to enhance absorption. Vitamin D has to be taken with fat because it's a fat soluble vitamin, not water soluble. The higher the dose, the more fat you need. So, if you're taking 10,000 international units, you need at least a tablespoon of fat like avocado or nuts and seeds. Dairy fat is not as effective. The calcium in dairy blocks your vitamin D absorption.

Are **B vitamins** important in menopause? Yes, but it's best to get your B vitamins from your foods – whole grains, legumes, and vegetables. Some women do not get enough vitamin B12 and folic acid. As you're going through menopause, you may not have enough stomach acid to convert vitamin B12 into its active form. Vitamin B12 and the activated form of folic acid are super important in the metabolism of your vascular system, neurological system, bones, and your detoxification pathways. You can get blood levels measured to be sure you're getting enough vitamin B12 and folic acid.

When necessary, I recommend the activated forms of these vitamins – methylcobalamin for B12 and methyltetrahydrofolate for folic acid – in a sublingual form, meaning underneath the tongue rather than orally. Most women who have issues with vitamin B12 and folic acid absorption are not going to absorb oral forms well from their gut, so we want to go directly into the bloodstream. The dose is 1,000 micrograms of each.

Women with anemia, genetic detoxification issues, or low blood levels, may need support. Measuring homocysteine levels in your blood can tell us if you're activating folic acid on your own. If homocysteine is high, you're not creating enough methyltetrahydrofolate and need supplementation.

Next is vitamin C, an antioxidant. **Vitamin C** is a water soluble vitamin like vitamin B, and women going through the change need more antioxidants in their diet. You can get an adequate amount of vitamin C by eating citrus fruits. Vitamin C is also found in red peppers and lots of different vegetables, but it's super easy just to squeeze some lemon or lime in your water and get vitamin C every day. Vitamin C can help reduce oxidative stress, which means you have too many free radicals floating around in your blood due to normal cell metabolism or high stress. Free radicals are very damaging to your heart, vessels, and the rest of your cells. Research shows that in menopausal women, oxidative stress decreases left ventricular function, the big part of the heart that pumps the blood throughout your body.

Vitamin C is important if you have osteoporosis, because it helps with bone health. The dose of vitamin C is 100 milligrams daily, which you can easily get in your diet. Some people use high doses – thousands of milligrams of vitamin C, which can flush out your colon and may cause a detox effect.

Vitamin E is often recommended for menopause and for women in general, because it seems to promote your hormones. Vitamin E is a fat soluble vitamin that acts like an antioxidant. There's only anecdotal accounts of the benefits of vitamin E for menopause symptoms, meaning that women report that they seem to be better taking 400IUs vitamin E to help reduce hot flashes. Again, I prefer you get vitamin E from your diet. One of the best sources are fatty foods like avocados.

Vitamin K is an important fat soluble vitamin that usually does not have to be supplemented. Vitamin K1 controls blood coagulation, and vitamin K2 maintains bone health. If you're eating green leafy vegetables, you are probably getting enough vitamin K1. If you're taking an anticoagulant or blood thinner like Coumadin, vitamin K1 can interfere with the drug. Your blood levels must be checked frequently on Coumadin, especially if you increase your intake of leafy greens.

Vitamin K2 is synthesized in your bone, meaning you actually make your own K2. Vitamin K2 is also synthesized by your intestinal microflora, but it binds to the flora so you don't absorb it well. Dietary sources of vitamin K2 include fermented soybeans, dairy products, egg yolks, and liver. Vitamin K2 impacts your bones in different ways. It regulates how your osteoblasts lay down bone, and also helps to form your osteoclasts, which are the cells that eat away old bone. Vitamin K2 works on both sides of the bone formation equation. If you have low vitamin K2 in your diet, you will have an increased risk of fracture. The dose of vitamin K is 50 to 150 micrograms per day. I usually supplement Vitamin K2 in patients who have osteoporosis.

Now, let's talk about **minerals**. Most of the minerals we consider for menopause have to do with prevention of bone loss or repairing bones. The majority of your bone is made out of calcium, and a small part of it is made out of strontium, phosphorus, and magnesium. Most of these minerals can be found in your diet. Unless you have osteoporosis or other specific health issues, I do not supplement with minerals.

Estrogens and drugs called bisphosphonates will slow your bone resorption and reduce bone turnover, but there's no drug that will increase osteoblast activity to grow bone. Only hormones – progesterone, testosterone, human growth hormone, DHEA – stimulate bone growth to increase bone density. If you are osteoporotic, then you need minerals in order to help increase bone density, but most of it is going to come from your diet.

Calcium is the major component of the bone. You need lots of calcium when you're a child so you can form healthy bones. Infants and young children absorb 60% of the calcium they consume in their diet – mostly from breast milk and dairy products. By the time you're in adulthood, calcium absorption decreases to 15-20%. The only time your absorption of calcium goes up is during pregnancy, because you need to absorb more, or the fetus is going to steal calcium from your bones.

You should be getting 1,200 milligrams of calcium in your diet per day and 1,500 milligrams if you have osteoporosis. The best sources of calcium are dairy products. For instance, a half cup of ricotta cheese has 335 milligrams of calcium. Greens are a good source, but you're going to have to have a whole cup of cooked greens to get 266 milligrams of calcium. Squeeze some lemon juice on your cooked leafy greens to help absorb the minerals.

You can also get calcium from fortified foods like coconut milk, oat milk, almond milk, soy milk, and orange juice. Eight ounces of these beverages usually have about 300 milligrams of calcium added. Another excellent source of calcium is eating fish that have bones, like sardines. A three ounce serving of sardines provides 325 milligrams of calcium.

If you drink a lot of caffeine, eat a lot of protein, or have a high sodium diet, you're going to excrete most of your calcium through your urine. If you drink a lot of caffeine or consume excessive amounts of alcohol, which affects vitamin D function, you will decrease your ability to absorb calcium.

In supplements, calcium is chelated, meaning it's bound to another molecule. Calcium carbonate is the most commercially available form, derived from shells and bones. These supplements should be taken with food because you need stomach acid to absorb calcium carbonate. A more absorbable form of calcium is calcium citrate, which can be taken with or without food. Minerals are usually chelated or attached to an amino acid. You'll find many different chelated calciums on the market.

If you are taking calcium as a supplement because you have osteoporosis, the maximum daily dose is 500 milligrams. If you take any more than that, you're just not going to absorb it very well. You must try to get the rest of the calcium from your diet. I have my patients take it with dinner because calcium can have a calming effect and help you go to sleep.

Another bone nutrient is silicon. **Silicon** improves your bone matrix and facilitates your ability to mineralize your bones. Bioavailable silicon is associated with denser bones and is found in whole grains, like cereals, quinoa, and oatmeal. Because it's made from grain, beer is actually a rich source of silicon. The dose of silicon found in supplements for osteoporosis is around 40 milligrams. Silica, a food additive, differs from silicon, and is not absorbed by your intestine.

Boron is a trace mineral that helps build bone as well. Boron is found in apples, almonds, avocados, bananas, broccoli, celery, pears, grapes, nuts, legumes, peaches, potatoes, prunes, raisins, and tomatoes. Boron is found in so many different plant foods that there should be no reason you're deficient. Boron can be found in osteoporotic mineral complexes at one to three milligrams.

Now let's talk about magnesium. **Magnesium** is an important mineral for bones, but also for cardiovascular and neurological health. Magnesium has a very calming effect, but if you take excessive amounts of it, it will cause diarrhea. That's because magnesium pulls water into your gut, which is how Milk of Magnesia works to make your stool softer. You have to be careful with the form of magnesium you're using and not take too much. Magnesium deficiency is very common in people who have gastrointestinal diseases like colitis, Crohn's disease, or celiac disease. Type 2 diabetics and alcoholics are often deficient in magnesium. And by the time you've reached your 60's, you don't absorb magnesium as well.

Dark chocolate is a great source of magnesium. Green leafy vegetables and legumes are also good sources of magnesium. Dairy products, nuts, seeds, and whole grains are also rich in magnesium. You can also get magnesium if your water is hard, but it's not the best source. Magnesium is added to fortified breakfast cereals and foods. The suggested dose of magnesium is 250 to 350 milligrams daily. If you're taking calcium, you need half the amount of magnesium compared to calcium. If you take more than that, you're more likely to experience diarrhea.

The last bone mineral is **strontium**. A trace mineral, 99% of your strontium is found in your bones. It's better to get strontium from your diet because if you supplement with strontium, it can replace some of the calcium in your bones. They'll be denser, but they won't be stronger. Seawater is rich in strontium, so it can be found in seafood and sea vegetation. Strontium can also be found in grains, leafy vegetables, and dairy products.

Other supplements

I use other supplementation to improve estrogen metabolism, particularly in cases of estrogen dominance, when you're making more estrogen than progesterone (like in perimenopause or premenopause), or you're taking hormone replacement therapy. Not every woman needs to improve her estrogen metabolism.

Some women have great estrogen metabolism. I find that my patients who are taking Genesis Gold® metabolize their estrogen fine. If my patients experience breast tenderness and bloating with their hormone replacement therapy, they may need some extra help. Estrogen metabolism tests can be ordered for high risk women to see if you're converting your estradiol into the safer form of estrone.

There are supplements I use to improve estrogen metabolism when you need extra help. These four food extracts work to affect your conversion of estrogen in a positive way, helping your body make more of the safe 2OH estrone, rather than the inflammatory 16OH estrone and 4OH estrone.

The first one is diindolylmethane or DIM. **DIM** is an IC3 indole – a compound extracted from cruciferous vegetables like broccoli, cauliflower, and brussels sprouts. IC3 indoles are the stinky, sulfur compound in cruciferous vegetables. The dose of DIM is 100 to 400 milligrams. However, lower is better. If you take too much, it may relieve your breast fullness and pain, but it may also induce hot flashes by blocking estrogen too much.

The second supplement, **isoflavones**, the phytoestrogens found in soy products and red clover, also improve estrogen metabolism. The dose is about 50 mg of soy isoflavones, and 40-80mg of isoflavones derived from red clover.

The third supplement to help estrogen metabolism are **flax lignans**, extracted from flax seed. The dose is about 600 milligrams a day of the extract. If you're taking ground flaxseed, you need 10 to 40 grams of ground flaxseed to get enough lignans to actually improve your estrogen metabolism.

The last supplement used to improve estrogen metabolism is fish oils, particularly eicosapentaenoic acid (EPA). **EPA** is one of several omega 3 fatty acids found in cold water fatty fish like salmon. While EPA helps to improve estrogen metabolism, in combination with DHA (docosahexaenoic acid) also found in fish oils, it has an antidepressant effect, especially when you're taking estrogen. EPA and DHA in fish oils may help regulate serotonin.

Fish oils help regulate inflammatory cytokines as well, to help decrease inflammation in menopausal joints. Fish oils and vitamin D are the most common extra supplements on top of Genesis Gold® that I use in my menopausal patients. I eat a lot of fatty fish, but find that if my joints are bothering me, taking extra fish oils can help.

Fish oils help reduce inflammation of the cardiovascular system too. Studies show that the higher the EPA to DHA ratio, the more reduction there will be in the CRP – cardiac reactive protein – an important inflammatory marker that indicates inflammation in your heart and blood vessels. In type 2 diabetics, a higher EPA to DHA ratio helps reduce triglycerides. Both EPA and DHA are important modulators of cell membrane function, helping tissues return to healthy homeostasis.

The dose is 1,000 to 2,000 milligrams a day, with a 2:1 ratio of EPA to DHA. If you take much more than that, you're just going to be belching up fish. Fish oils are better taken with food because you need stomach acid, induced when you eat, to help absorb fish oils.

I also like to make sure that my patients are getting an adequate amount of **probiotics**, both for their colon health and their vaginal health. Maintaining a healthy colon is vital to help absorb nutrients from food. And if your colon is healthy, you will have a healthier vagina, because you're going to have more lactobacillus. When you're premenopausal, your estrogen promotes your vagina to colonize with lactobacillus. Lactobacillus metabolizes the glycogen stored in vaginal cells to produce lactic acid, which helps maintain a healthy acidic vaginal pH. That's why it's called lactobacillus acidophilus.

A low acidic pH inhibits your vagina from growing other pathogens, because other microbes from your colon can colonize your vagina, including E. coli, Enterobacteria, Candida, and Gardnerella. If you have enough lactobacillus acidophilus, it won't allow those other microbes to overgrow. Probiotics in your diet positively affect the microflora of the vagina, which can help with some menopausal vaginal symptoms. Adequate probiotics can help prevent infections which are common when you're postmenopausal because you have a very alkaline pH. Insuring adequate levels of vaginal lactobacillus helps prevent vulva-vaginal candidiasis or yeast infections, as well as vaginosis, which is an overgrowth of other bacteria.

Probiotics are in Genesis Gold® because I don't think most of us get enough probiotics. We don't eat enough fermented foods to get the probiotics that we need, so there is a variety of probiotics in Genesis Gold® to help support your colon and vaginal health.

Probiotics are taken orally, so lactobacillus migrates from your colon to your vagina. If I have a patient who has chronic vaginal infections, especially in the postmenopausal period, I will have her add lactobacillus acidophilus in powder form into her estriol vaginal cream, and use it for a week or two to help recolonize her vagina.

To help assist my menopausal patients with insulin resistance and weight gain, I recommend berberine. **Berberine** works by upregulating the cellular energy switch called AMPK (adenosine monophosphate protein kinase). In fact, berberine is as effective as the drug Metformin to reverse insulin resistance and help you lose weight. It also helps lower blood lipid levels and improves your liver's glucose metabolism. Berberine is more effective than metformin at reducing your waist circumference and waist-hip ratio.

This is why I recommend that you ditch your scale and start with body measurements. Your goal is to lose inches, especially around your waist. You can plug your body measurements into an online calculator to calculate your body fat percentage and pounds of lean body mass. The goal is to maintain or increase your lean body mass and lose body fat.

The recommended dose of berberine is 500mg with each meal. But you must go slowly to avoid gastrointestinal upset. Start with one per day with lunch for up to a week, before adding a second dose for up to a week, then add the third dose. You must be sure you're eating a real meal with balanced carbohydrates, fat, and protein, or your blood sugar may bottom out.

Common side effects of berberine include stomach upset and nausea, which is why you need to titrate your dose up slowly. Rare side effects are rash (due to sensitivity to berberis alkaloids) and headache (possible due to low blood sugar and alkaloid sensitivity). Berberine can rev up your metabolism, so get your body used to it by starting it at lunch, not dinner, or it may interfere with sleep.

Berberine cannot be used long term. I recommend only three months of use. If you're supporting your hypothalamus with Genesis Gold®, then your weight loss will not disturb its homeostasis, and you'll be able to maintain the weight loss.

Since brain fog is such a common issue in menopause, another supplement I recommend to help improve memory is CDP-choline. **CDP-choline** is an essential intermediate in the pathway of the phospholipids that make up your cell membrane. In your brain, it helps nerve cells transmit information. Your body naturally makes CDP-choline, but with age and poor diet, you may not make enough. While CDP-choline works in the brain, it also helps cells all over your body. When taken by mouth, it is absorbed almost completely.

CDP-choline is beneficial to your neuroendocrine system, so it helps to improve the communication between your nervous system and your hormones. It helps to modulate your neural-immune system, meaning decreasing brain inflammation, and it also has neurophysiological effects, improving the way your nerves fire to carry vital messages.

Studies on CDP-choline show that it's neuroprotective in hypoxia ischemia. This means that if you've had a stroke, or you've lost oxygen to the brain due to trauma, it can help to protect your brain. CDP-choline is used to heal traumatic brain injury. While there have not been studies in humans on CDP-choline for learning and memory, we see clinical improvement in patients' memory. I've used it myself in times of high stress, and it works very quickly to boost memory if you're providing your brain with the nutrition it needs, which I get from taking Genesis Gold® daily. The dose of CDP-choline is 250 to 500 milligrams for brain fog.

Alternative Therapies

Let's talk about other alternative therapies that you don't swallow. These interventions can be used in addition to making sure you get your hormones properly balanced with hypothalamic support. Rather than taking drugs and multiple supplements, you can use these therapies.

The first category to help treat menopause symptoms are **mind-body interventions,** including: hypnosis, cognitive behavioral therapy, biofeedback and relaxation training, mindfulness-based stress reduction, and yoga.

Hypnosis seems to decrease hot flashes subjectively, meaning a woman feels like she experiences fewer hot flashes. And objectively, when monitors are placed on the subject's skin, women have 57% fewer hot flashes. Hypnosis also seems to improve self-reported sleep quality and sexual function.

The next mind-body intervention is **cognitive behavioral therapy** (CBT). CBT includes education, motivational interviewing, relaxation, paced breathing, and different strategies to improve your symptoms. Studies show CBT may be beneficial in reducing hot flashes and other physiological symptoms of menopause.

What about **biofeedback and relaxation training**? This technique uses biofeedback to train your body into progressive muscle relaxation. Thermal control biofeedback, meaning measuring the temperature of your skin, and training you to pace your respirations to induce relaxation, can be helpful. Relaxation recordings can be used at home to help menopausal symptoms. There has been some research to show some of these techniques actually work pretty well.

Relaxation training may work because when there's elevated sympathetic activation of your nervous system, meaning your nervous system is hyped up, it causes you to have more vasomotor symptoms, which include hot flashes, trouble sleeping, and anxiety. These techniques can help to relax you and allow those symptoms to be lessened. Studies using progressive muscle relaxation with slow deep breathing significantly reduced both objective and subjective symptoms of hot flashes compared to controls. But even just paced respiration, meaning pacing your breathing and slowing it down can significantly reduce hot flashes.

A therapy that I do personally and teach to my patients is a relaxation technique using conscious contraction and relaxation. If done right before you go to bed, you may sleep more deeply and decrease night sweats.

Here's how you do it:

Consciously contract your body in a wave from your toes to your face. Very slowly, contract your toes, feet, legs, buttocks all the way up, taking very slow, deep breaths. When all of your muscles are completely contracted, stay like that and hold your breath for a few seconds. Then very, very slowly release the contraction, again, from your toes back up to your head, relaxing every muscle in a wave. Breathe deeply. Repeat the contraction/relaxation cycle three times. This technique has been shown to induce GABA by increasing your parasympathetic nervous response and lowering your sympathetic nervous response. As a result, it will reduce hot flashes and night sweats, and induce deeper sleep. If you wake up in the middle of the night, it's a great exercise to help get back to sleep.

Another mind-body technique is **mindfulness based stress reduction**. Mindfulness based stress reduction uses a variety of exercises like mindfulness meditations and yoga to develop awareness and acceptance of the present moment. So many times, we're worried about the future or worried about what happened in the past that we're not in the present, and we feel anxious. Mindfulness based stress reduction can help teach you to be more present. It has been found that by practicing these techniques, hot flashes seem less bothersome subjectively, but objectively, there are not significant improvements in the vasomotor symptoms of menopause. While we really need a lot more studies in this area, I do believe mindfulness is a great practice to help you be calmer, which can help your transition through the change of life.

Yoga falls into the mind-body intervention category. There is moderate evidence for the short term effects of yoga on the psychological symptoms of menopause. This means that when you're practicing yoga over a short period of time, you may experience less anxiety, depression, or stress. But it hasn't shown improvement in vasomotor symptoms, like hot flashes, or somatic symptoms, like vaginal dryness. Nonetheless, yoga is a great way to become present in your body, and it's great for stretching and keeping aging joints and muscles limber.

Whole System Alternative Medicine

The second category is called **whole system alternative medicine**. Unlike conventional, or allopathic, medicine, which separates the body into different systems – so you see a gynecologist, a cardiologist, and an endocrinologist, for example – these alternative medicine systems look at your body as a whole. I'll be going over the alternative medicine approaches that have been studied in treating menopausal women.

Reflexology is a type of massage on your feet and your hands. The principle behind reflexology is that you have acupressure points at the bottoms of your feet and on the palms of your hands that correspond to certain body zones. When pressure is applied to those points, it's believed that energy blockages which may be causing disease can be released.

There are only a small number of controlled studies that look at reflexology, and the findings are very inconsistent, but patients do report that having a reflexology treatment helps them feel calmer. Reflexology may be something to explore.

Homeopathy is another alternative medicine approach. Homeopathy is the principle that "like cures like." In allopathic medicine, which is conventional medicine, we use something different to cure a symptom. For instance, if you're having a histamine reaction, like itchy, runny nose and eyes, an antihistamine drug is used. In homeopathy, you would use a histamine-inducing homeopathic dilution to treat the histamine reaction. The dilution is such that you don't even find the herbs in the homeopathic solution, just the energetic vibrational imprint, which seems to work fairly well in certain incidences.

I use homeopathy as part of my personal medicine chest. Some 30 years ago, while visiting relatives in Hawaii, my husband had a severe allergy attack. He usually treated these with high doses of antihistamines, but nothing was working. So the kids' Yiayia (Greek for grandmother) suggested we go to a natural health store, where we found a homeopathic remedy for his allergies. Surprisingly, it worked really well. Since then, I've been playing around with homeopathy for certain symptoms. I say "playing" because I'm not a trained homeopathic health care provider. While I have not found homeopathy to be super effective for menopausal symptoms, I do use it for other types of issues.

What about **acupuncture**? Acupuncture is a treatment used in traditional Chinese medicine. It involves inserting tiny needles into your skin at certain points on the body. These acupoints are along meridians, through which energy runs in the body. The foundation of belief is that diseases and symptoms occur because there's disruption in your Qi, which is your life force, or your energy. There's been a lot of study on acupuncture for various menopausal symptoms. Some research shows no significant difference between acupuncture and placebo needling of non-acupressure points. Other trials do show that acupuncture improves sleep and somatic symptoms more so than placebo. I have used acupuncture for inflammatory conditions like pain, and it's worked well, but I have not used it for menopausal symptoms.

And then there's **traditional Chinese and East Asian medicine.** A lot of my patients will try this type of medicine. Traditional Chinese medicine includes Chinese herbs, massage that you do on yourself, acupuncture, diet, and meditative exercises like Tai Chi. The modalities are usually tied together, and are based on your Qi being interrupted, which is believed to cause disease. There is some evidence that traditional Chinese medicine may be effective in relieving menopausal symptoms, but the findings are mixed overall.

The problem is, like most alternative therapies, they're rarely used by themselves. Most complementary alternative medicine modalities are used in combination, so it's hard to do research on them. Unless you're just doing acupuncture, or just doing massage, or just using essential oils, or just doing meditative exercises, though if not combined with other modalities, they are not as effective. It's hard to actually find single modalities that are effective. If combining modalities works for you, then that's what you may need to do.

If you're interested, these alternative treatments like mind-body techniques and whole system medicine are worth giving a try. I am not promoting any of these for menopause, because I haven't seen that they've worked alone for my menopausal patients. With the exception of certain Chinese herbs which may cause kidney damage, most of these therapies are safe and worth a try. Please be sure you have good functioning kidneys before taking Chinese herbs.

The Foundation of Treating Menopause

What do you use as a foundation, or something that you can build upon that will address the root imbalances induced by going through the change? I just presented a lot of modalities to use in menopause. What I do instead for my patients and myself is use hypothalamus support. By supporting your hypothalamus, you provide the vital foundation to optimal functioning. The rest of the therapies, including hormones, can be used to help mitigate symptoms.

If you have osteoporosis, you may need to take some extra minerals and bone support. If you have an estrogen metabolism issue, you may need to take some extra DIM or flax lignans. Treatment is according to your particular issues. However, I always recommend starting with hypothalamic support.

I created Genesis Gold® for the hormonally challenged, and there's no one more hormonally challenged than a woman going through the change. We miss our hormones. When they start to fall, everything becomes havoc in our system.

Let's explore how Genesis Gold® works for the change. The main ingredients in Genesis Gold® are the Sacred Seven® amino acids, uniquely blended to support your hypothalamus. You're not going to find that precise blend anywhere else. The non-GMO plant-derived amino acids help to support hypothalamus function, and work best in combination with all the phytonutrients that are in Genesis Gold®. Genesis Gold® helps to keep your brain healthy, your moods more stable, your energy more abundant, your sleep deeper, and it helps to balance your hormones. If you need extra support on top of Genesis Gold®, I recommend adding extra Sacred Seven® for a short period of time, about three to six months.

Genesis Gold® is rich in whole plant foods and sea vegetation to provide the micronutrients necessary to help rejuvenate aging cells. The phytonutrients in Genesis Gold® that help with graceful aging include fennel, flax, royal jelly, maca, ashwagandha, licorice root, lemon peel, and fo-ti. These were particularly chosen to improve hormone receptor sites, enhance your collagen production, improve your skin texture, and strengthen your lean body mass so you feel younger and healthier. Genesis Gold® helps support healthy metabolism, cellular metabolism, as well as estrogen metabolism. The ancient sprouted grains in Genesis Gold® provide the phytonutrients necessary to support cellular metabolism and enhance mitochondrial energy production.

The phytonutrients also support age-reducing telomere lengthening. Telomeres are at the end of your DNA. When telomeres are longer, you are biologically younger. When telomeres are shorter, you're biologically older. The grape seed extract in Genesis Gold® particularly works to increase telomere lengthening, and antioxidant pomegranate seeds and broccoli sprouts which are rich in DIM, help to improve safe estrogen metabolism. I don't take extra estrogen metabolism support because I've been taking Genesis Gold® for a long time with my hormone replacement therapy. I'll only take extra DIM if I drink more than one glass of alcohol and have breast tenderness.

I included immune optimizing phytonutrients in Genesis Gold® like maitake, reshi, Pau D'Arco, suma, tumeric, garlic, olive leaf, and astragalus. You want protection against infection and cancer, yet the micro-dosing of the Genesis Gold® herbal extracts helps calm down your hypersensitive menopausal immune system. When you go through menopause, and especially in the postmenopausal period, your immune system can be hypersensitive, so you'll have more allergies. There seems to be less hypersensitivity in my menopausal patients who take Genesis Gold®.

Because menopause adversely affects your gut, I designed Genesis Gold® to help optimize your digestion and detoxification. Genesis Gold® has prebiotic artichoke, and a variety of beneficial probiotics, as well as ginger and betaine, which is a natural form of hydrochloric acid, apple cider vinegar, and pancreatic enzymes that help to improve your menopausal digestion and absorption of nutrients. Beet root and sunflower lecithin help improve liver detoxification.

Since it was manufactured in 2003, Genesis Gold® seems to enhance cell receptor site activity, so my patients need much less hormone replacement therapy.

Optimizing the function of your hypothalamus with Genesis Gold® can help you thrive through the change of life.

ACTION ~ What alternative therapies might you be interested in using as part of your Menopause Action Plan?

Part Five

Packing for the Trip

Chapter 11

Pillars of Healing

Whether premenopausal, perimenopausal, menopausal, or postmenopausal, I help my patients focus on five pillars to heal. These five pillars focus on hypothalamic healing to balance hormones, improve neurological and immune function, and help menopausal patients live their best lives. This is everything you need to do when you're in menopause. It's really important that you pay attention to all five of these pillars. If you're just focusing on one, and not the other four, you're not going to thrive.

I know change is hard. When we do go through a shift, it's often easier to tackle one change at a time, and that's fine. It usually takes a minimum of two weeks and up to 40 days to set a habit. So you can work on one pillar at a time, and then work on establishing the next good habit. After a few months, you'll have it all dialed in. It's going to be easier if you take a frank look at your particular lifestyle in regards to each one of these five pillars, and ask yourself: "Is this aspect of my lifestyle as healthy as it could be so that I can really thrive during the change?"

Pillar #1 Your Nutrition

We are what we eat. If you put junk into your body, your body doesn't have much to work with. By junk, I mean trans fatty acids, fried foods, fake sugars, fake fats, and foods that have been contaminated with pesticides and herbicides. These foods are void of essential nutrients, so your body is not going to get the nutrition it needs to heal. Plus, it's going to be working overtime to get rid of the toxins you're feeding it.

If you have a very limited diet, your body will not get the variety of nutrients it needs to heal. It is not enough to live off a handful of supplements and eat a crappy diet. Your diet is the foundation of nourishment your body needs in order to heal.

Now, I absolutely believe that supporting your hypothalamus during the change with Genesis Gold® will help fill in nutritional gaps, but it will not make up for the standard American diet. A diet of white flour, white sugar, high saturated fats, trans fatty acids, excess red meats and devoid of fruits and vegetables will not provide the nutrient foundation you need to survive the change. There's research that shows that what you eat while you're going through the change affects your symptoms as well as your health.

A study looked at dietary patterns in 400 Middle Eastern women suffering from pretty severe menopausal symptoms. The researchers found the dietary pattern that was associated with the least amount of symptoms was the pattern where the women ate the most fruits and vegetables. The dietary patterns that had the most symptoms like hot flashes, insomnia, and moodiness, were either full of fake food, or mostly using plant-based oils like mayonnaise and vegetable oils, or super high in saturated fats and sugar. Neither of the junk food dietary patterns included enough fruits and vegetables.

In that same study, the researchers added up all the antioxidant capacity within the dietary patterns, including co-factors like vitamins B, C, A, and E, as well as coenzyme Q10. These micronutrients act as antioxidants to get rid of oxidation in your body, which is the natural waste effect of your cells making energy. Oxidation creates free radicals that cause cellular and tissue damage. The more antioxidants you have in your diet, the better. The researchers found that the higher the antioxidants were in the fruit and vegetable pattern diet, the fewer menopausal symptoms these women had.

In another interventional study, 17,000 menopausal women were instructed on how to eat. Their hot flashes were measured before and after the year-long study. The women who ate more vegetables, fruit, fiber, and soy had a 19% reduction in hot flashes. That doesn't sound like that much, but if you're suffering pretty badly and you add these foods to the other pillars I'm going to talk about, it's going to make a big difference.

Does dairy have a place in menopause? Well, actually, it does. In a study looking at 750 postmenopausal women, the ones who ate the most dairy and animal protein actually had higher bone density than the ones who ate the least. These women had a higher level of vitamin D and calcium intake, as well as a 17% reduced risk of going through early menopause.

What about eating grains in your diet? A study of 11,000 postmenopausal women found that those who were eating 4.7 grams of whole grain fiber in a 2,000 calorie diet compared to 1.3 grams of whole grain fiber had a reduced risk of early death. So fiber from a plant based diet makes a huge difference in your health.

What are the healthiest fruits and vegetables? They're all good for you. But for proper hormone metabolism, focus on cruciferous vegetables, which are rich in the IC_3 indole DIM. One study found that women who ate the highest amount of broccoli had decreased levels of 16OH estrone that was linked to breast cancer and farmore protective 2OH estrone. Your diet should include at least 3-4 servings a week of cruciferous vegetables: broccoli, cauliflower, brussels sprouts, and kale. You can roast, sauté, or eat them raw.

Dark berries have been found to be incredibly beneficial for women going through the change. An eight-week study was done on menopausal women who consumed 25 grams of freeze dried strawberry powder daily, and the researchers found that the women's blood pressure was lower. Multiple studies have demonstrated that berries – blackberries, mulberries, blueberries, cranberries, boysenberries, raspberries, and pomegranates – have so many antioxidants that they lower the inflammatory markers in your blood, and help to reduce your risk of heart disease.

So how do you put this all together? I have a lot of patients who come to me, and they're just eating in pieces. They may add a handful of berries into their regular diet, or a bunch of broccoli, or a little soy. Yet, they really need to adjust their overall nutritional plan, and their overall dietary lifestyle.

If you could adopt any lifestyle diet out there, which one has the lowest risk of mortality and chronic illnesses like cancer, heart disease, diabetes, and will actually help you through menopause?

The lifestyle diet that has received the highest ratings for years is the Mediterranean diet.

The Mediterranean diet has the greatest adherence, meaning it's the easiest to follow. It's the healthiest diet to reduce the risk of obesity, including becoming overweight in menopause. The Mediterranean diet provides a better cardio-metabolic profile, meaning you're less likely to have inflammation and cardiovascular disease, and it helps to improve menopausal symptoms.

The Mediterranean diet is so healthy because it's plant based. Over 50% of the calories come from vegetables, whole grains, legumes, and fruits. For optimal health, your body needs lots of micronutrients –

vitamins, minerals, antioxidants and phytonutrient cofactors – that are found in plant foods.

Second, the Mediterranean diet is naturally rich in healthy fats, with 30% of the calories coming from fat. Specifically, this diet has lots of anti-inflammatory monounsaturated fats like olive oil, which help your body create healthy cell membranes and receptor sites to allow hormones into the cells.

Third, the Mediterranean diet includes lean protein. Protein breaks down into amino acids, and which your body needs to heal and keep biochemically and hormonally in balance. Fifteen to twenty percent of the calories in the Mediterranean diet come from protein.

So what does the Mediterranean diet look like?

The foundation of the Mediterranean diet is plants – mostly vegetables, whole grains and legumes. Your hypothalamus loves it when you're eating lots of plant foods, because this tells your hypothalamus that the environment you're living in is healthy and bountiful. Daily intake of whole grains, olive oil, fruits, vegetables, beans and other legumes, nuts, herbs, and spices is crucial to helping you thrive during the change.

While you can get protein from plant sources, the Mediterranean diet also includes animal sources, like eggs and dairy, usually through cheeses and yogurts, as well as fish and fowl, but very little red meat. Animal flesh is limited to just once a day.

Olive oil is the primary fat. Other foods naturally containing healthy fats are highlighted, including oily fish like salmon and sardines. Avocados and nuts are also included. Monounsaturated fats like olive oil are incredibly anti-inflammatory, and provide your body with the fatty acids necessary to help create not just hormones, but also hormone receptor sites and healthy membranes.

Olive oil is used for cooking, and to dress foods. Drizzling olive oil on grains, vegetables, and proteins helps to get enough of this super healthy fat in your diet. Plus, cooking with olive oil maintains the nutrients in foods better than any other oil.

The biggest issue I see with my patients and students who are going through the change and want to clean up their diet is they really need to learn how to cook in a healthier manner. The majority of us learned how to cook from our family of origin. If you grew up on a diet that was not healthy, or too heavy in starch, fat, or sugar, you tend to adopt those taste preferences and cooking habits. I'd like to challenge you to learn how to cook healthy meals, because it is absolutely key.

When I first started my Hormone Healing Circle, which is a circle of women who are really dedicated to healing themselves, one of the biggest issues was that they wanted to eat better, but they just didn't know how to cook. One of the things I did for this group was create videos to teach them how to cook some of the basic foods that I was trying to introduce to them. This training made such a big difference - they began posting pictures of what they had cooked in the support group and reporting how much they loved vegetables cooked this way. They even found that their families learned to like these vegetables too.

Something else I did for this group and for my patients was develop a nutritional plan to help them make the best dietary choices. When I recommend they follow a Mediterranean diet, they still get really confused. They get confused because they're used to counting calories. I want them to pay attention to macronutrients and learn what is a fat, a protein, or a carbohydrate.

Many of my overweight patients. and those with specific health issues, need to know how many grams of fat, protein, and carbohydrates they need each day. So I created my version of the Mediterranean diet – my DMAR Nutritional Path to Healing. It's a really great guide to know exactly what your body needs for each of the macronutrients. I'm going to gift it to you at the end of this book.

What about water? Water should be your main beverage. I prefer you drink filtered water. You can add lemon or lime juice to your filtered water if you'd like to make it a little tastier. You need to drink one ounce per kilogram of your body weight per day. So if you weigh 130 pounds, that's 60 ounces of water.

Some people actually drink too much water, and oftentimes, it's because they're not getting enough salt in their diet. Many of my patients clean their diet up so much that they don't put any salt or spices back in, so they don't get enough electrolytes to absorb the water into their cells. So they're constantly drinking way more than they need. You may need to add a little salt in your diet, preferably sea salt for trace minerals. I like to vary my sea salt. Himalayan salt is also good. And for taste and extra micronutrients, I use lots of spices and herbs.

What about caffeine? I was not a coffee drinker before I was premenopausal. Then, one of my patients who really couldn't afford to see me had a coffee shop, so we bartered. Being a police officer, my husband was a coffee drinker, especially before his shifts, so we got our money's worth in coffee for him. Because of this, I learned to like coffee. Drinking coffee actually slows me down. I tend to be the kind of person who jumps up in the morning and starts my day like a bulldozer. I drink coffee in open ceramic cups that'll break, so I actually sit down with my coffee and enjoy it.

Coffee reminds me of my grandmother and my husband's grandmother who made drinking coffee a ritual. They'd drink a little bit in the morning, and they would drink a little in the afternoon when they would sit down from their chores and just relax. To me, drinking coffee is a way to relax.

Mayo Clinic found that the more caffeine you drink in postmenopause, the more problems you'll have with hot flashes and night sweats. On the other hand, in perimenopausal women, caffeine improved their mood, memory, and concentration. Caffeine enhances your arousal, your attention, and your mood. Remember, take everything in moderation. If you're using caffeine to wake up in the morning or in the afternoon to get a little boost, you need to consider that your adrenals may not be functioning optimally.

What about alcohol? Data from the Nurses Health Study was very interesting regarding alcohol consumption. Beginning in 1976, the Nurses Health Study has involved hundreds of thousands of women, and is still going on. The researchers found that the death rate in the 35 to 59 year old age group was lowest in women who were light to moderate drinkers, compared to heavy drinkers and nondrinkers. More than two drinks per day is considered heavy drinking.

The more alcohol you consume, the lower your bone density becomes. Alcoholics have very low bone density because alcohol interferes with vitamin D absorption, as well as vitamin D processing in the liver. Breast cancer rates also increase with heavy alcohol consumption. So you need to pay attention to your alcohol intake. A glass or two of wine with dinner, preferably red wine rich in polyphenols, is healthy. Three or more glasses could be a problem.

On occasion, if you drink more alcohol than you should, consider taking some DIM to help metabolize the alcohol into a safer form of estrogen. If you're using alcohol to calm down, you really need to learn alternative stress reduction techniques. Remember, everything is fine in moderation.

Crazy strict diets are not healthy in menopause. You should be adopting a healthy nutritional lifestyle that becomes the way you eat all the time. Consuming fruits, vegetables, legumes and whole grains, restricting processed foods, and drinking more water all makes a huge difference in your health all the way through the change.

One of the reasons I've not suffered from severe menopause symptoms is I was raised on the Mediterranean diet. My mother was Italian, and never adopted the American way of cooking. We always had lots of vegetables, very little red meat, lots of fish, and some poultry. We didn't drink milk, but did eat yoghurt and cheese. Mom was a great cook, and used lots of Italian spices and herbs. She taught us to sauté and roast, but she never fried our food. My sisters and I were introduced to vegetables very early, and they were prepared well so we made them part of our diet. It's never too late to change your taste buds. Work on it by eating a healthier diet now, even if you're postmenopausal.

Pillar #2 Your Activity

Being active throughout your life helps to reduce your risk of chronic illness. Regular exercise will help you maintain a healthy weight. It'll relieve stress, reduce the risk of disease, and improve the quality of your life. Studies that have followed postmenopausal women for 12 weeks of regular exercise report positive change in their vitality and mental health.

The biggest effect of exercise is on your cardiovascular system. Regular exercise decreases blood pressure and improves the tone of your heart. There's a balance between the sympathetic nervous system, which gets you going, and the parasympathetic nervous system, which calms you down. In the heart, this balance is called vagal tone, where the two aspects of the autonomic nervous system activate the sinoatrial node in your heart to keep it beating. If you have a nice balance between your sympathetic and parasympathetic nervous system, you have good vagal tone. If your vagal tone is off because you're not exercising regularly, you're going to have more problems as you reach the postmenopausal period. Vagal tone has nothing to do with hormones, but it has to do with aging.

Just like you lose tone in your skin and muscles as you age, you lose tone in your heart. However, postmenopausal women only have poor vagal tone while resting. When they exercise, if they're in good shape because they've been exercising since they were premenopausal, their vagal tone is just like a woman who's not in menopause. Good vagal tone means you're fit. Loss of vagal tone is one reason you may experience heart palpitations when you're at rest. During postmenopause, you may notice that your heart feels like it's racing a little bit or skipping beats when you're lying down. You almost never feel them when you're running around, exercising or doing chores.

Heart palpitations can begin in perimenopause because your estrogen levels are falling, and you're losing neuroendocrine communication that helps direct your heart. Will age-related loss of vagal tone kill you? Absolutely not. Keep fit and your heart will keep you healthy. Studies show that premenopausal and postmenopausal women have identical heart rates and good vagal tone when they're exercising. But postmenopausal women have a little less vagal tone when they're resting and after exercise.

Exercise increases your cardiopulmonary function. If it's done regularly, at least a few times a week, exercise will help increase your good large particle HDL, reduce the bad small particle LDL, reduce triglycerides, and reduce fibrinogen, a molecule in your blood that contributes to blood clots.

Regular exercise reduces high blood pressure, and decreases the risk of heart attack and stroke. Plus, regular exercise creates a calorie deficit, meaning you burn more calories, so it can help minimize weight gain during the change. Menopausal weight loss is not just about dieting, but it's about keeping active as well. You have to burn those calories too. Regular exercise increases your bone mass, especially strength training and impact activities like walking or running.

Swimming and cycling are great for your heart, but do not create the impact that stimulates bone growth. Exercise can offset bone loss and prevent osteoporosis.

Exercise also can reduce lower back pain, which becomes an issue as you get older and lose core muscle tone. Without core muscle tone in your abdomen, and back and hip girdle, your vertebrae are not well supported. Because of this, they become unevenly stacked with less space between them. Your vertebral discs, the little gel filled sacs that keep your vertebrae apart, lose fluid with age and flatten, causing nerve impingement. Your muscles work harder to keep your spine in alignment, which becomes painful. Stretching and core exercises help keep your back healthy.

Exercise also helps to reduce stress and improves your mood. Exercise may also help reduce hot flashes and improve sleep because it balances out your sympathetic and parasympathetic nervous systems. When you exercise, you have a less over-stimulated sympathetic nervous system and a calmer parasympathetic nervous system. Sedentary people have a much more active sympathetic nervous system, which increases hot flashes and interrupts their sleep.

What is my recommendation for exercise going through the change? First of all, don't start anything new without having a complete physical and making sure it's okay with your healthcare provider, especially if you have heart disease, arrhythmias, a recent heart attack, or uncontrolled blood pressure. If you're basically healthy going through the change, the recommendation that I'm going to give you is going to make a big difference in maintaining your lean body mass, gaining cardiopulmonary fitness, and actually reducing your chances of getting chronic illnesses.

There's three aspects of exercise: aerobic exercise, strength training, and flexibility training. Fitness is a three-legged stool, so you need to do all three types of exercise.

Aerobic exercise gets your heart rate up. You need to be aware of your target heart rate, which will be about 60-70% of your maximum heart rate. Your maximum heart rate can be calculated by subtracting your age from 220. For example, if you're 50 years old, your maximum heart rate is 170. Your aerobic target heart rate is 102 – 119. If you are a heart patient, you need to check with your doctor on what target heart rate is safe for you.

An easy way to track the intensity of your exercise is to use the talk test. Exercise becomes aerobic if you're moving fast enough that you cannot keep up a running conversation. If I'm exercising alone, I sing to myself. When I can no longer sing out loud, I'm in the aerobic zone. If you're walking with a friend and able to talk, that's not aerobic, you need to walk faster or go up hills. You want to exercise fast enough so that you can't keep up a running conversation without catching your breath. That's aerobic.

You need two and a half hours per week of aerobic activity. You don't have to do aerobic exercise daily. Three days a week is sufficient to keep your heart healthy and your body fit. Any aerobic exercise will do - rowing, cycling, swimming, dancing, walking, running, hiking, surfing. Any time you're exercising and breathing hard, you're getting aerobic activity.

What about strength training? According to your particular health issues, there are different recommendations for strength training. Women with osteoporosis build bone faster if they do very heavy weightlifting, but only one set. You should work with a trainer to be sure you're doing it safely.

Strength training can come in a lot of different forms. You don't have to go to a gym and lift weights. You can do yoga or Pilates. You can do exercises using your own body weight, like push-ups, sit-ups, and tricep dips. You can use exercise bands that provide resistance to strengthen your muscles. There's lots of ways for you to do strength training, but you've got to make sure that you're working on all parts of your body – your legs and buttocks, your back and stomach, your arms and shoulders. Strength training one to two times a week will help keep you strong and fit.

Every day, you need to stretch. The third leg of the exercise stool is flexibility. Older people are more likely to get hurt because we lose our flexibility with age. Joints and muscles stiffen up. Without focusing on flexibility training, you're more likely to hurt yourself when you're active and exercise. You always want to warm up before you stretch. You can use a hot shower, hot bath, or a jacuzzi to warm your muscles before stretching. I like to do aerobic activity and then a little stretching.

There's lots of different ways that you can incorporate these exercise recommendations. If you need to lose weight or you're diabetic and your blood sugar is out of control, you can do High Intensity Training (HIT). What I have been recommending for my patients for many years now and do myself is a simple HIT routine.

First you warm up for five to seven minutes with an aerobic activity – walking, running, swimming, cycling, rowing, dancing. Then do a 20 second burst of speed followed by one to two minutes at your warm up pace. That's one interval. Do three intervals before cooling down for five to seven minutes.

The whole HIT routine takes 17 to 20 minutes to do, and can be done just three times a week. HIT can reduce hemoglobin A1C, get your blood sugars under control, and your cholesterol levels balanced, so you're making more protective HDL and less of the unhealthy LDL. HIT can also help get your weight under control. This HIT routine is fast and simple.

Then once a week, I recommend a long slow distance (LSD). Exercising at a slower target heart rate (less than 60% of your maximum heart rate) for over an hour can help you burn body fat for at least 48 hours. LSDs can increase your endurance to keep up with your busy life. Plus, hiking, long bike rides, and walks are stress reducing.

Now, strength and flexibility training should also include balance training, which is super important, especially if you have osteopenia or osteoporosis, because you want to prevent falls. If you're going to go hiking, use some trekking poles. I do recommend light bouncing to help increase bone density. You can use a trampoline or you could skip rope. A little bouncing for about five minutes every day helps to stimulate bone growth.

Remember that fitness requires **aerobic**, **strength**, and **flexibility** training.

Pillar #3 Your Sleep

The third pillar for healthy hormones in menopause is getting an adequate amount of deep sleep. Now, I know it can be hard to sleep when you're going through the change. Your declining hormones affect your sleep, but there is so much you can do about your sleep environment to induce deeper sleep. First, after dusk, don't use any digital devices. Your hypothalamus directs your pineal gland's production of melatonin. If you're looking at a screen on your phone, tablet, computer, or television after dusk, you're telling your hypothalamus it's still daytime. The blue light from these screens is the same light waves as daytime. So your hypothalamus doesn't trigger your pineal gland to make melatonin.

If you must be on screen after dusk, blue light blocking glasses can help. Of course, you're still getting stimulated by what you're watching on the screen. Especially if you're consuming disturbing news before you go to bed. That kind of stimulation is going to get your sympathetic nervous system revved up, and you will not be able to fall asleep. So no digital devices after dark, and no disturbing news. That's number one for your sleep hygiene.

Try to establish a bedtime routine. That could be a bath or aromatherapy. I like to put some essential oils in my bath with magnesium salts to make it really relaxing. You can also read or journal to calm down. Maybe you have a beauty routine that you do every night that helps you to relax and fall asleep. Think of these 15-30 minutes as me-time.

If you can, go to bed at the same time every night to help establish a healthy circadian rhythm. And then, you need to have all of your lights out. Your room needs to be completely dark. If there are street lights shining into the room, get blackout curtains. This also means that no digital lights should be in the room. Those little blinking lights are going to interfere with your sleep quality. You may not feel like you're awake, but you're not going into deep sleep when your skin is perceiving those lights. Even putting an eye mask over your eyes isn't enough if that light is on your skin. Many patients will tell me it's hard because their partner likes to watch TV before they go to bed, and then falls asleep with it on. That is the worst thing you can do if you want a good night's sleep. I believe TVs in bedrooms interfere with deep sleep. Watch television in a different room. You shouldn't be on those digital devices after dusk anyhow.

The temperature of your room affects your sleep. If it's too hot, you will not go into a deep sleep. In order to make melatonin, you need a cool room temperature between 60 and 67 degrees Fahrenheit. Breathing in cool air while under a nice cozy comforter will help deepen your sleep. Room temperatures over 70 degrees interfere with deep sleep.

Then, get up with the sun. You want to establish a healthy circadian rhythm. If you're sleeping in late, you're going to bed too late. Try to get up as early as you can around the same time every morning to establish a healthy circadian rhythm by telling your body the difference between day and night. Try to avoid taking naps during the day. If you're regularly napping during the day, you're going to have a much harder time sleeping at night. A lot of people tend to want to take a little afternoon siesta as they get older. It's fine to relax, but napping messes up your nighttime sleeping.

Be sure that you're active, but don't exercise after dark. Exercise is stimulating. You make cortisol to fuel your exercise, which interferes with melatonin production. So it's going to be harder to bring yourself back down into nighttime mode. Be sure you're exercising during the day – the earlier the better – and stay active during the day. Get up and move around if you're sedentary. If you have a sedentary job where you're sitting for hours, make sure that you get up and move around every hour for at least for 10 minutes.

Pillar #4: Your Mindset

Your mindset determines your healing. Thankfully, your mindset is not inherited. It's learned, so it can be unlearned. You can change your unhealthy mindset into a healing one.

Did you know that you can boost your immune system by positive thinking? I can't tell you how many times I've walked into a room of a patient who was sick – coughing, sneezing, spewing out germs. Before I walk into the exam room, I tell my body, "This is not my bug." And I can count on one hand how many times I've gotten sick from another person in over 30 years. I talk positively to my body and nurture a healing mindset.

In order to successfully navigate your menopausal transition, you must adopt a healing mindset.

Studies show that your attitude towards the change will determine your experience. Your attitude is influenced by cultural norms. What does your family believe? What did your mother and your grandmother believe about menopause? Did they think it's a good thing or a bad thing? If your belief system is, "When I go through the change, everything is going to fall apart. I'm going to lose my beauty, my health, my vitality," you're setting yourself up for a bad experience. If you've been raised to feel that going through the change is a gift, and say, "I've lived this long, this is great, I've made it, now I'm the wise woman in the family," you're going to have a much better experience during and after the change of life.

Besides your past, your present environment affects your mindset. If you're under a lot of stress presently, it's tougher to go through the change. Humans tend to be afraid of change. But once we're through it, we actually shift. Menopause is going to happen to every woman. It will happen to you if it hasn't already. So it's all a matter of being prepared for it with a healthy mindset.

Research proves that negative beliefs held prior to menopause predict a more difficult time going through the change. Your mindset begins in your youth. If you had a negative attitude towards your periods, you will have a more negative attitude towards menopause, not seeing it as a positive natural event. And you're more likely to have more issues in menopause. Changing your negative thoughts and attitudes results in a reduction of your symptoms.

If you're premenopausal now, make friends with your period, and learn to appreciate your body. Start to make that shift mentally now, because it'll make menopause so much easier. Studies show that women with negative attitudes tend to be younger and premenopausal, but postmenopausal women tend to have more positive attitudes towards menopause. Why? Because postmenopausal women have lived through it, and realize they've survived.

That's one of the reasons I waited to write this Menopause Action Plan book. I wanted to be through my own menopause, and get to the other side of it to show you it's survivable. Not only can you survive, but you can thrive.

By the time you're going through the change, you might have some unhealthy coping mechanisms from your youth or adulthood, and now they're being exacerbated in menopause. For instance, if you've used alcohol to cope, you may find you're drinking more. Or maybe you're a shopaholic, and you're spending too much money.

We all have issues, and if we haven't dealt with our core issues when we're going through a shift, the change may bring them up to be healed. Just be more mindful and present, and pay attention to when you're using unhealthy coping mechanisms, and how they're not really helping you through this transition. This is an opportunity to see that you need to make changes regarding those coping mechanisms and adopt healthier ones.

Here are some keys to help shift into a healing mindset.

First, practice stress reduction techniques. Stress reduction techniques are definitely part of mindset training. More importantly, stress reduction techniques help reduce your experience of stress.

Learn deep breathing techniques, meditate, and practice mindfulness. You need to adopt a technique that suits you and helps you learn how to reduce your stress reaction. I know it's hard to shift your mindset without changing your reaction to stress. If your knee-jerk reaction is to get freaked out, practicing these techniques will help calm you. If you're a worrywart, it may be hard to unlearn, but it's possible.

I have seen women in mid-life go from being super worried and very reactive to stress, to learning how to calm down and be less reactive. The change changes the way they deal with life. They become a calming influence for everyone around them.

Stressors will not stop while you're going through the change. In fact, they tend to multiply and intensify. Perhaps you're going through the change with children and parents who depend on you. Plus you're working. You have a lot on your plate, and your hormones are all out of balance. And it's tough learning stress reduction techniques and practicing them. It's great to know how to meditate, and how to deep breathe. But if you don't do it on a regular basis, it's not going to help. When you practice these techniques consistently, you actually train your body to respond to stressors in a positive way.

I developed a CALM meditation to help my patients and students. It's an exercise that uses deep breathing, and integrates scent and sound. The limbic system in your brain controls your emotions, and your stress response is triggered by scent and sound. In this CALM meditation, you teach your body to make GABA using scent and sound while deep breathing. Deep breaths stimulate the parasympathetic nervous system, which induces GABA production to calm you down. If you associate deep breathing with a scent and sound, and you're in a troubling stressful situation, all you need to do is hum a little bit of the sound to yourself or smell the scent, and your body automatically makes GABA.

I will gift you with my CALM meditation at the end of the book.

When you go through the change, you actually change. You start to realize what's really important. You stop being so reactive to the small stuff. That's one of the gifts I've experienced going through my own menopause. What I was reactive to when I was younger was a lot of small stuff that just doesn't bother me anymore. For instance, I'm not such a neat freak as I used to be. The house doesn't have to be perfectly clean because it's not that important, especially now that I have my toddler granddaughter running around the house.

When I had my own toddlers, it stressed me out when they got fingerprints all over my glass coffee tables. I didn't realize that it was more important to appreciate the time with my babies. There's definitely been a shift in my own mindset with age. I see this in other women as they get older and realize what's really more important.

Another way to shift your mindset is to practice positive thinking. I know this sounds kind of cliché, but there are studies to show that it's not necessarily your negative thoughts, but the absence of positive thoughts that have the greater impact on your health and wellbeing. We all have negative thoughts, such as when we think, *oh my gosh, this is killing me.* Immediately reverse it with a positive thought like *this is making me stronger.*

If you don't ever have any positive thoughts, your body is just listening to what you're saying, and that may actually kill you. Practicing positive thinking means you start introducing positive thoughts. One of the best ways that I've found to do that is to keep a gratitude journal. I record what I'm grateful for at the beginning of the day before I get out of bed, and again before I go to bed at the end of the day. Writing it down forces me to think about those positive things. There's a lot to be grateful for. Gratitude has been shown to rewire your brain so that you create a shift in your stress response and your mindset.

With positive thinking, if something bad happens, I may immediately have a negative thought because it's a reflex. Then, I follow that with a positive thought, and if I can't think of anything positive, I ask myself, "What can I be grateful for in this moment?"

In my early premenopause days, I learned how to look for the gift in a situation, right in the moment. It's easy to see the gifts in any negative situation after it's passed. Perhaps something horrific happened ten years ago. It may be easy to see why it happened, what you learned from it, and what was positive in your life after this transformative event. Yet, to be able to find the gift in the midst of the chaos is key. And as you go deeper through the change, I guarantee that by the time you're in postmenopause, you're going to have it nailed. You're going to know exactly what the gift is in every situation.

People in your life will be looking to you for guidance, saying, "This awful stuff is happening to me right now, what do you think might be good? Is there anything I should be focusing on because I just can't see it?" And you'll be able to see it. You'll be able to help them see it. More importantly, you're going to be able to see the gifts in your own daily life if you're practicing stress reduction techniques and positive thinking.

A third technique to help shift into a healing mindset is to laugh. Do as much as you can to induce laughter. Laughter stimulates your immune system. Laughter enhances your learning and memory. It helps you cope better with the stressors in your life. Watch funny shows, play games, or sing silly songs. Just laugh, because it changes everything. Studies on the immune system show that laughing triggers natural killer cells and T-cells to go after cancer. Laughter is incredibly healing.

Then, I want you to find time to practice me-time. Make time for yourself. When women actually make themselves a priority, even just 15 minutes a day, dramatic changes occur. If you incorporate, let's say, relaxation techniques in your day and that becomes your me-time, it's going to increase muscle relaxation, quiet your mind, promote positive emotions, learning, concentration, creativity, and reduce some of your symptoms. You are worth the time, so carve time out of every day for yourself. Even if it's just five minutes to keep your gratitude journal, that's me-time. Taking that relaxing aromatherapy bath at night to sleep better, that's me-time.

Appreciate me-time. It's just not another chore. Learn to love this time. Realize that if you don't spend that time on you, you're not going to be good for anyone else in your life. It really makes a difference when you focus on yourself. Your exercise is part of your time, but find something you really like. It could be a hobby that becomes part of your me-time. It could be a different thing every day that becomes your me-time, but make sure you carve that time out of your day, or the stressors of life will catch up with you. You won't be able to shift your mindset if you don't spend some time with yourself.

Next, I want you to practice presence. That means staying in the moment, and being mindful, aware, and present at each and every moment in your life. Being present prevents you from worrying about the future or dwelling on the past, and it brings so much joy.

The biggest gift I've found in entering the postmenopausal phase is that I notice that I'm spending more time in the present moment, and much less time in the past and the future. I know that sounds kind of crazy, and very new age. But honestly, the key to happiness is being present in the moment. What is happening before you right now is more important than anything else. Now, I get in a bit of trouble about this because I have surrounded myself with protectors who tend to be worrywarts. When I'm super present in the moment, like taking my toddler granddaughter out on a bike ride, and forgetting to call when we're running late because we've spent way too much time with the chickens and the sheep that we saw all along the way, it'll worry my husband. I tend to be so present in the moment that time escapes me. So, yes, check in with your loved ones, but stop and smell those roses.

The last thing that is so important to shifting your mindset is staying connected. Your social support is key to your health, and can help you live longer. We know that people who live alone tend to die earlier than people who live with other people, whether they're still married, or they live with extended families, or in residential care and get to do things with other people. Social support is key.

Your friends are part of your support. Your children and grandchildren are part of your support. Your partner or spouse is part of your support. One of the things that we forget as we go through the change, especially if you're partnered with someone close to your age, is that they're probably going through their own change at the same time. Studies show that in heterosexual couples who've been together a long period of time, male hormones actually shift right along with their female partner's hormones. When women are younger and cycling with periods, their male partner's hormones follow along with hers. As she starts to decline in perimenopause, so does he. As she reaches menopause, he goes through andropause, which is the male version of menopause, and means making less testosterone. I've seen the same phenomenon in my same sex couples. We reflect one another hormonally.

We're sharing similar experiences in a different way. We may have different ways of coping. One way of reconnecting with your partner is to start dating again. If you've been going out on dates since the beginning, great. But if you don't date regularly, you need to start. Taking the time to check in with each other, especially during this part of your life when things are changing, can heal and strengthen your relationship. By dating, I mean do something together that you both enjoy, not just doing your regular chores or eating together like you regularly do. Do something a little bit different. Be sure to talk in this special time together, share your feelings, and reconnect. It'll make everything about your life better, including your sexual relationship.

Sometimes, sex can become a little bit stale when you've been with the same partner for a long time. You're both changing, and maybe you don't have as much interest in sex. Maybe you're not as juicy as you used to be. Yet, now you're starting to use hormones and supplements and supporting your hypothalamus with Genesis Gold®, you're getting a little bit juicier. You've got to get to know each other again. Sexually, things are a little bit different, and orgasm can take a little bit longer. So you need to learn to be intimate differently together. This could be a great adventure. Many of my postmenopausal patients say that sex is better than ever. It's great because they have better communication with their partner than when they were younger. This is a shift in your mindset. Perhaps you're not as concerned about how you look, but more about how you feel. And that makes everything better.

There's a change in your relationships, with your spouse, your children, your grandchildren, your friends, but you may still need more connection. You need to find your pack, your circle of women. Other women going through the change with you. Women who choose to make this the best time of their life. They may be your friends, or perhaps women outside of your circle of friends who can help you navigate the transition in a much healthier way.

Finding women who have a similar philosophy about menopause with whom you can talk about what's happening and find the gifts can be incredibly helpful. It's one of the reasons that I started my Hormone Healing Circle, because I believe women need circles that they can go to for support. In days gone by, women had knitting circles or quilting circles. They would get together and talk about what was going on in their lives. We've lost a lot of that type of activity, so we need to find some kind of circle with other women where we can discuss what's happening in our lives and support one another. This is especially important during the change.

Pillar #5 Support Your Hypothalamus

The fifth pillar of your healing to thrive during the change is supporting your hypothalamus. Your hypothalamus controls your metabolism, your sleep, your memories, your moods, and just about everything vital in your body. If you support your hypothalamus through the change, and the earlier the better, it helps you to thrive. It helps you to not just survive the change, but actually thrive. I have seen major mindset shifts in women who are going through the change when they take Genesis Gold®.

When I first dreamt of the formula to heal the hypothalamus, my intention was to help heal us physically, emotionally, mentally, and spiritually. Since Genesis Gold® has been available, I've actually witnessed some incredible mind-body-soul healings. I've watched as patients and customers shift their mindset from one of victimhood to healing, to one of suffering through symptoms, to optimizing their life and making changes necessary to be whole.

With the help of Genesis Gold®, women who had the most difficulty shifting their diets, exercise programs, or even sleeping habits have been able to make those changes. Their mindset starts to shift, and they start to believe in themselves. They start to realize why they were keeping their weight on, or doing all the work for others and not for themselves, and start to find out what's important for them. When they become happier, everybody in their life becomes happier.

It's key that your hypothalamus gets the support it needs, and it's hard to do it with diet alone. I've been eating a healthy Mediterranean diet almost my entire life, yet it still wasn't enough to keep my hormones in balance.

Once I started supporting my hypothalamus with Genesis Gold®, everything got into better balance – I experienced healthier hair, nails, skin, and was aging much more gracefully. My symptoms of menopause have been so much less than what I've seen in my own family members. More importantly, I've experienced a mindset shift towards deep appreciation of what's most precious in life. Now I'm able to share this information with women like you who are going through the change so you too can thrive.

ACTION ~ What lifestyle changes are you willing to make in order to thrive during this change?

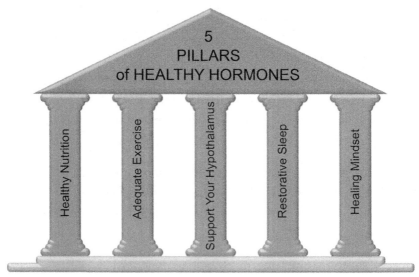

Chapter 12

Empowered Menopause

Now that you understand where you are in the change, what's happening to your body, mind, and soul, and most importantly, what you need to do to treat your symptoms and age gracefully, it's time to partner with your healthcare provider so that you get the care that you need.

This chapter is all about empowered menopause. Learning to speak up for yourself, getting what you need, and taking control of your life is part of becoming empowered.

What does empowered menopause look like?

I want you to imagine yourself feeling happy, beautiful, strong, and sexy. Yes, you are all that. And the world reflects your amazing self right back to you. People want you to share your wisdom. You're living your best life. You're thriving. This is truly possible when you are empowered going through the change.

What does it look like to thrive during menopause? Not just surviving and getting rid of all your symptoms, or working on your wrinkles and losing that weight, but what's it like to actually thrive? I have a few stories to share with you before we jump into working with your healthcare provider. Becoming empowered in your personal life will allow you to step into empowerment when partnering with your health care provider.

Empowered menopause is the key to living your best life.

These are women who began menopause just like you. They struggled and suffered with symptoms. They shifted their mindsets about menopause. Each woman had a different Menopause Action Plan. Now they're each living their best lives and making a difference in their worlds.

The first story I'd like to share with you is about a woman who I treated about 20 years ago. Let's call her Michelle. Michelle was going through the change, and wanted to talk about hormone replacement therapy.

Michelle was a little concerned because she had issues in her family with different kinds of cancers, but we determined that she was probably at a fairly low risk, as long as we were doing the screening tests. So she started on bioidentical hormone replacement therapy. Michelle held a powerful position for a pretty big company, and had learned to be successful in a man's world.

Once she started using bioidentical hormone replacement therapy, and then started supporting her hypothalamus with Genesis Gold®, Michelle shifted. She became a lot more feminine. She stopped wearing pants as often, and started wearing flowing skirts. Michelle even wore her hair differently. She started to indulge in a neglected hobby, and began painting again. Michelle was spending more and more time with her art, to the point where she felt like she could make a living doing what she loved. So she retired from her position and became an artist, and is now very happy.

Research shows that women often change their careers when they reach menopause. Women over 50 are actually very good at making the shift to something more fulfilling, because they have a lot of life experience. Of course, it's difficult to make those changes when you're hormonally challenged, moody, have brain fog, and are struggling with all your symptoms. Yet once you get back into balance, there are a lot of opportunities out there for you.

After 50, your interpersonal skills are very well developed, so careers working with people are well within your grasp. Potential positions could include a real estate agent, financial advisor, working in the healthcare field as a nurse, occupational therapist, personal trainer, tutor, counselor, or even personal chef. If you're not happy with the career you're in now, this is a great time for you to make a shift to one that will truly fulfill you.

I met Charlotte when she was well into postmenopause. Charlotte struggled in the beginning of menopause, choosing not to use hormone replacement therapy, but remedied herself with botanicals. In spite of her struggles, Charlotte embraced the change as an empowered time. She retired from teaching, and moved into grandmotherhood. This woman is probably one of the sweetest, wisest sages I've ever met. Charlotte teaches others, particularly women in her community. Her gift to the world is supporting others at the spiritual level, especially postmenopausal women.

Denise is a lawyer, and went through menopause really early, but did not get the help she needed. Her doctor did not believe that she was going through the change, even though she was sweating and couldn't sleep through the night. Her weight had ballooned up to 170 pounds. She called herself an out-of-control mess. Her doctor insisted that she was too young to go through menopause, but she insisted on blood work, and it showed that her FSH was high.

Denise was definitely menopausal, so she started to see me. When a new patient comes to see me, I'm pretty thorough about examining them. She got a full exam, extensive blood tests, and even a stool evaluation. I inquired about all of her daily habits, her work life, her sex life, and her spiritual life.

You may think this isn't part of going through the change, but it is. I'm sharing this with you because you deserve to work with healthcare providers who will inquire about all aspects of your life. You are more than the woman sweating before them. You have a life that is being affected by the change. You have a job. You have relationships. You have habits that might need to shift. You have a sex life if you choose. You have a spiritual life. All aspects of your life are affected by the change.

I started Denise on a rather intense regimen of supplementation, including Genesis Gold®. I also prescribed her bioidentical hormone therapies. She began with quite a bit of supplements to heal her gut, but we gradually decreased all of it as her body responded. She continues to take Genesis Gold® and bioidentical hormones. Within a year and a half, Denise looked 15 years younger. Her weight was down to 128 pounds. She was no longer sweating, and she slept well. She had a healthy sex drive and enjoyed her life. Denise said people couldn't believe how much energy she had. She even had enough energy to run for mayor!

You too have the opportunity to make menopause a stepping stone into a whole new way of being. It's your choice. But first, you've got to get the help you need. It's so important that we, collectively as women, and especially those of us who are healthcare providers, normalize menopause. It isn't a disease, and there's nothing to be ashamed of. And we as women need to cast off our fear about treatment, and feel empowered enough to seek the help that we need.

Some interesting studies have shown that the phenomena of menopause in its experience leans more on the threat to our feminine identity, and less on the latent opportunity. Meaning, we're more concerned about who we are as women because our worth has been associated with our youthfulness and our reproductive years, and less on the opportunity presented by the change. It's time that we redefine our feminine identity and retrieve ourselves, in order to become who we truly are.

Research has found that women felt they were losing their femininity as they went through the change. They feared being different from what they were always expected to be, and they didn't have support. They didn't have enough support at home. They didn't have enough support from other women in their lives. They didn't have the support they needed from the health care community.

Going through the change is a time in which we can redefine our feminine identity and shift our self-image. It's moving from just surviving menopause to a full acceptance of the change. It's a time to embrace it wholeheartedly to actively and effectively cope with your menopause, whether it's with hormone replacement therapy, supplementation, or mind-body stress reduction techniques.

Your wisdom is shifting. You are gaining peace of mind. You have the time to do soul retrieval, and retrieval of your true self. This is an opportunity to seek advanced empowerment and become a truly empowered woman. You need to be active in your own self-care. You need to practice mind-body techniques to actually be the boss of your body.

I envision myself as a rider on a horse. My body is the horse, and my soul is the rider. In my younger years, I was just hanging on for dear life, because my soul wasn't in control. As I went through perimenopause, my soul became one with my body. Now, I'm riding in this graceful bliss that I just didn't have when I was a younger woman.

As an empowered woman, you can move towards the treatment of your choice, because you feel that sense of empowerment to effectively partner with your healthcare provider. Empowered women going through the change guarantee that their health is robust.

You have to choose what is best for you.

Since I became a nurse in 1983, I have championed the idea of being your own best advocate. Shortly after graduating from UCLA, I gave birth to my first child, who was born intersex, with lots of medical issues.

My baby's issues were so profound that the medical community had no idea what was best. Before I became pregnant, I'd had a dream of a blond haired baby boy. My baby was born with ambiguous genitalia and XY male chromosomes. At the time, the doctors' recommendation for babies like mine was to surgically remove the testes, create a vagina, and raise them as female.

Intuitively, I felt that was wrong. My baby needed to be raised the way they wanted to be identified. So, empowered by my maternal instincts, I went against medical advice. But I had to fight the healthcare system. We were in an HMO at the time, which was very difficult to navigate, even though I had a nursing degree and did all my research on what to do about this child with so many endocrine issues.

My firstborn is why I do what I do, and why I became the "Hormone Queen." I had to learn about hormones to save my baby. Yet, I wondered how people without any kind of medical training navigate the healthcare system on their own. When I became a nurse practitioner, right before I gave birth to my daughter, my main goal was to teach people how to be their own advocates. First, I had to become an advocate for them, then teach them how to be their own advocates so they could get the healthcare they needed.

We focus on relationships with other people – your significant other, your spouse, your children, your parents, your friends, your coworkers. It is now time for you to establish an effective relationship with your healthcare provider. Do you feel like you have a partner in your healthcare provider? A lot of women don't. They only see their health care provider when they have an issue. They don't go to set new goals, or prepare for potential health issues. They don't go with a plan.

You have a unique opportunity to partner with your healthcare provider because you have your own Menopause Action Plan.

You know exactly what you need. You've made your choices, and now you have a plan to bring to your healthcare provider. It's time now to partner with them so they can help you the best way that they can.

Studies show that most patients, women in particular, favor evidence-based, individualized risk information and shared decision-making, leading to informed choices. What does that mean? It means you want to know the evidence behind the treatment choices, and you also want a personalized therapeutic plan. You want to be looked at as an individual. You want your health care provider to notice what your risks are as an individual, not assume everyone else's risks are yours and limit your treatment choices. You want to share in the decision-making process so that all the choices you make are truly informed.

The study demonstrated that the discussion of risks would be optimized if the provider offered unbiased, truthful, summarized information, and also personalized the risk information and treatments for menopause, especially regarding hormone replacement therapy. In other words, women don't want to be given the same thing that every other woman in that practice is given. They want what is best for them, and they want their treatment personalized. Women want to know what their potential personal risks are, and what they can do about them.

So why doesn't this happen enough in healthcare? Studies show that around the world, women are not able to really work with their healthcare providers effectively. There are known barriers preventing effective partnership for both healthcare providers and their female patients.

What are the barriers preventing healthcare providers from working with you?

One barrier is that healthcare providers just don't have enough time. Trying to see too many patients limits the time needed to get a complete history from a patient, examine them, and educate them. In the United States, the average length of doctor appointments are less than 17 ½ minutes. For half of the world's population, primary care doctor visits last less than five minutes. That's not enough time.

My first consultation with a patient lasts two hours. We explore their entire history, their present life, their spiritual life, their sexual life, their work situation, environmental exposures, and all of their risk factors. We talk about everything needed to develop their personal Menopause Action Plan.

We talk about their goals, and all their symptoms. I spend a lot of time educating them on what's happening in their body, and what their treatment options might be, so they can make the best choices for themselves. It takes time, and the follow up visits are usually 30 to 45 minutes, sometimes up to an hour to go through everything that we've been working on and make sure they're doing well with the treatments they have chosen. Lack of time is the number one barrier your healthcare provider has to working with you.

The number two barrier is that oftentimes, healthcare providers don't have the best communication skills. Early in college, tests are often given to students, which help determine their skills and interests to guide them towards appropriate career paths. Physicians are lined up along with engineers and contractors, while nurses are lined up with pastors, counselors and teachers. People who are attracted to nursing tend to have better communication skills than people who are attracted to medicine.

It's one of the reasons I chose to become a nurse practitioner – to really help people. I did not want to only view my patients through the lens of pathophysiology. I wanted to see their potential for optimal wellness – physically, psychologically and spiritually. I found that the best way to help people is by being able to communicate with them, educate them, and support them. You have to find a healthcare provider who will listen to you and communicate what you need to know in a language that you can understand.

Studies show that the lack of consistent communication in the healthcare system leaves women unknowledgeable or misinformed about menopause and all its related issues. Inaccurate information concerning a health-related experience that every woman will undergo has negative implications for women, their healthcare practitioners, and the entire society.

The third barrier is that healthcare providers often have a lack of empathy. They may be an empathetic person, but if they haven't lived through the situation themselves, it is difficult for them to feel genuine empathy.

Almost thirty years ago, I had a Jamaican patient whose experience was a good example. At the time, I was working in a gynecological practice with a male gynecologist who loved to do surgery while I did most of the counseling and education. This woman had just had surgery and had come to me to talk about sex. I asked her why she wasn't seeing the doctor. She said, "Because he keeps referring to it as marital relationships. I have a relationship with my mother, I have a relationship with my postman. It's not a marital relationship issue. It hurts to have sex now. I need him to be able to say the word sex so I can communicate with him, and since he's uncomfortable, I'm here with you."

If you feel comfortable enough to talk about the fact that your vagina is dry and sex is painful, or you're not orgasming, or your brain is so foggy that you cannot remember your grandchild's birthday, but your healthcare provider can't speak your language, you have an issue. Most women prefer to work with a female healthcare provider, especially one who's maybe a little ahead of them in the change in order to have some kind of shared experience.

The fourth barrier that healthcare providers have to developing an effective partnership with you is they may not be open to your choices, especially alternative therapies. Part of the problem is their fear of malpractice if they don't treat you with conventional protocols.

You might be asked to sign off if you want bioidentical hormones, because there aren't studies on bioidentical hormones like there are on pharmaceuticals, nor are there big pharmaceutical companies that you can sue if you have a problem with the hormones. So healthcare providers can be afraid of liability. That's why it's important for you to have complete informed consent, meaning that you understand the risks and you agree to the treatment.

Women are not only seeking alternatives to conventional pharmaceuticals. They're seeking alternatives to conventional care, where their menopause experience is solicited, their treatment goals are heard, and they are engaged as agents in managing their own menopause. That's what I want for you. I want you to manage your own menopause, and partner with your healthcare provider. It's a two-way street.

What are your barriers to communicating effectively with your healthcare provider?

Studies show that lack of knowledge or misinformation about the change can be a barrier for you. But guess what? You just finished reading the Menopause Action Plan. You have educated yourself about exactly what's happening in your body, what your risk factors are, and what your choices are.

The second barrier is not knowing your options. Many women go to their healthcare provider and say, "Okay, I'm having these issues. Just give me what you've got," and walk out with a prescription.]But that's not true for you, because you now know your options – both conventional, like hormone replacement therapy, as well as alternative options. Hopefully at this point, you know what the best options might be for you, and if they require a prescription, like hormones, you can get what you need from your healthcare provider.

The first two are not barriers for you anymore now that you've completed your Menopause Action Plan. But number three might be a barrier, and that's believing that your healthcare provider knows your situation better than you do. When this happens, you give away your power.

Giving away our power is a very common barrier, because as women, we oftentimes have a tendency to defer to authority. In our mothers' and grandmothers' generation, doctors were considered gods, so if they said, "Take this pill," you took the pill, and you didn't ask questions. That's not true anymore. You have access to so much information. You can look up every prescription that's offered to you, and look at all the risk factors and all the benefits and make your own choices.

Your healthcare provider doesn't know better than you about your situation. However, they are your best partner at getting what you really need so that you can take care of yourself through the third book of your life. It's time for you to become your own best advocate.

Let me share with you the techniques I use to help empower my own patients.

Perhaps you may want to look for these in your own healthcare situation. See if this feels good for you.

The very first thing that my patients do before they even get an appointment is they interview with my trusted assistant to be sure that they're really ready to do the work required to meet their healing goals. Being ready, able, and willing is key to your success.

While I love working with my patients, I don't see myself as their savior. I see myself as their partner. I can't go home with them and make sure they're eating well, exercising, meditating, communicating their needs to their spouses, using their hormones, and taking their supplements. I have to trust them. And they have to be ready, because there will probably be some lifestyle changes that need to be made, and it's going to take some work on their part.

So they go through a little interview process to make sure that they're ready, because it's an investment of their energy, time, and finances. I want them to be super successful. Once they arrive in my office, I do a couple unique things.

First, I don't wear a lab coat. I stopped wearing a lab coat when I was taking care of pediatric patients, because a lot of them were afraid of the lab coat. I only wear it if I'm doing a procedure that might make my clothes messy. I don't wear a lab coat with my adult patients because I don't want to induce white coat syndrome, which may raise their blood pressure from being anxious.

Second, I sit very close to my patients. There's no desk between us. I literally sit knee-to-knee with them. The reason I sit so close is because oftentimes, we are talking about very personal things, and I rarely have a woman who consults with me for the first time who isn't brought to tears. It's because she comes to some deep realizations about what's happening in her life. She feels a sense of hope and it's quite emotional. And those tears are good tears, they're healing tears. So we have lots of tissues in the office.

I also like to sit close enough to touch my patient on her knee, hand, or shoulder to demonstrate that, "I'm here for you. I hear you. I see you." Compassionate listening is key. In the beginning, it's a lot of listening and asking the right questions to help discover what I need to do to help them.

A very significant question I ask each of my patients is, "What's preventing you from reaching your health goals?"

Sometimes, they reply, "I don't know enough about the change." Or, "I don't really know what's going on." Or, "If I only had the hormones I needed..." But by the time we start really discussing what's going on in their life, they often realize that what's preventing them from reaching their health goals is them. They are not as empowered as they could be to make effective changes. They're not doing everything they need to do to make the shift. They don't truly believe that they can heal. Their answer to this question is a big eye-opener for them.

I share stories relevant to their situation to help patients open up. Sometimes, you're not really sure what to even ask. I have the gist of what's happening before you come in for a consultation, because you've created a beautiful narrative by writing down everything you think is going on. We'll talk about your situation and your concerns, and then if I suspect there's more you're not telling me, I'll share some stories. By hearing somebody else's story, you may realize, "Oh my gosh, that's like me." And that helps you open up a little bit more.

I also demonstrate my teachings. I'm a fan of drawing out your body systems and biochemistry on big pieces of paper. I used to draw it out on the protective white paper that's on top of the exam table, but my patients would want to take it home. So years ago, when my mother used to be my business manager and run my practice, she got big sheets of paper for me to draw on. Most of the time, my patients are so hormonally challenged when they first see me, that they have trouble remembering everything. So it helps them to have these tangible teaching tools, like bringing the chalkboard home.

I also provide them with educational materials that I've created – diets and exercises and information about hormones and recommended supplements. And my patients leave with my recommendations in writing so they know exactly what they need to do to begin healing.

Plus, I give out a lot of hugs. I'm a true believer that hugs are healing, and I've rarely met a patient, male or female of any age, who by the time we're finished is not open to ending with a hug.

Years ago, when I was the president of the California Coalition of Nurse Practitioners, we were working with the Nurses Service Organization, which was an organization that provides malpractice insurance. However, they did not cover nurse practitioners like me who had their own practice. The trend was growing, so I was trying to show them that nurse practitioners in solo practice were a safe investment liability-wise.

We were scheduled to meet after I was done seeing patients, so they were in my waiting room, watching what was going on. When we finally met in my office to talk about malpractice risk, they said they had never seen so many hugs given out. My patients got hugs from me as their healthcare provider. They got hugs from the medical assistant. They even got hugs from my mom who was running the practice and checking them out. The Nurses Service Organization had done studies on practitioners and found that those who had physical contact with their patients had far more trust from their patients. Human connection is important in any partnership.

I also provide my patients with avenues for accountability. I give them a lot of things that they need to do in order to heal. It's hard to make so many changes without support, so they get access to support groups. These are online because I have patients from around the world.

Besides access to online support groups, patients have different options to communicate with me. They are able to email, text, or call with questions. We offer in-person, phone, and video conferencing appointments. I've been providing telemedicine since 1999 before it was called telemedicine. All these options allow them to be able to check in when they need to, and help them stay accountable.

Like my own patients, my goal for you is that you become your own best advocate.

How do you get your healthcare provider to help you?

Remember, it's a partnership. You're at an equal level. That's why I sit right in front of my patients at the same level. I'm not above them, below them, or standing over them with a chart or computer, taking notes. I'm sitting at the same level because we're partners.

First, you need to know what you need from your healthcare provider. I'm going to give you my recommendations for all the screenings, as well as the blood work that I believe you need from your healthcare provider to get started in this partnership. Remember, you're coming in with your Menopause Action Plan completely filled out, so you know exactly what you need, but you still need some things from your healthcare provider in order to be sure that you're as healthy as possible, or, if you're having some issues, that you get some screening done.

Number one, you need a full exam from head to toe every year. Head to toe, meaning not just a gynecological exam. I do this for all my patients of all ages, all genders. As you get older, it is very important that your healthcare provider examines all of you – your heart, lungs, abdomen, ears, nose, throat, neck, lymph nodes, skin, scalp, joints, muscles, nerves, breasts and, of course, a thorough pelvic exam, including a rectal. I examine everything, even posture, because someone may think their symptoms are part of menopause, and it could be a structural issue. You deserve a full head-to-toe exam every year.

What about a pap smear? You should have a pap smear every three years if you're in a mutually monogamous relationship, meaning you're only having sex with one person and that one person is only having sex with you. If you're not in a mutually monogamous relationship, or if you've had abnormal paps in the past, then you need one every year. If the pap smear is abnormal, we also run Human Papillomavirus DNA because HPV is the most likely cause of cervical cancer. I'll also do STD testing at that time if necessary.

I do a yearly urine analysis on every patient. It's a quick look for potential diabetes, liver issues, and bladder infections. If they're complaining of any vaginal issues, I may do a wet mount, looking at their vaginal discharge under a microscope to make sure that there's no bacteria or fungus, and that the cells look healthy. All of this is done in my office.

My patients leave with a requisition for blood tests. The blood tests that I recommend for all women going through the change are: Follicle Stimulating Hormone (FSH) on day three to five of your cycle if you're perimenopausal, any time of the month if you're menopausal, or postmenopausal. A luteinizing hormone (LH) only if you're menopausal, as it doesn't make sense to do it in perimenopause unless you're concerned about fertility.

I'll order testosterone if you're complaining that your libido is low, or if you have bone density issues and are menopausal. I do a full thyroid panel – TSH (thyroid stimulating hormone), free T_4, and free T_3. I need all three to evaluate if there's a hypothalamus-pituitary-thyroid axis issue. I look at the adrenals by measuring DHEA-S (the active sulfated form of DHEA), and may order an expanded test if it's low.

I'll order a comprehensive chemistry panel that looks at electrolytes, kidney, and liver health. I do this because you're more than just breasts and a uterus – we need to look at your whole body. Plus, if you're coming in with a satchel full of supplements and medications, I want to make sure that there's not any damage to your liver or kidneys.

I also order a complete blood count with differential. Differential means that I'm looking at all the types of white blood cells to make sure you have a healthy immune system. In my older patients who have low white blood cell counts, I'm concerned about them eventually developing cancers because they don't have the white blood cells to fight it off. If you have allergies, you may have high eosinophils. While I'm a hormone specialist, I also deal with allergies, because as a family nurse practitioner, I look at you as a whole person.

I do a full lipid profile and measure particle sizes. Remember, when we talk about LDL and HDL particles, bigger is better. I do a high-sensitivity cardiac reactive protein (CRP-HS), that tells me if you have systemic inflammation. If CRP is high, even with a low cholesterol level, you're more likely to have a stroke or heart attack.

I'm looking for those metabolic markers to make sure you don't have inflammation. I look at hemoglobin A_{1c}, and depending on the patient, I may get a C-peptide. Both provide information about your glucose metabolism to be sure you're not insulin resistant.

I measure a prolactin level between 8:00 and 9:00 a.m. If your prolactin level is too high, it will block your hormone receptor sites. So if we give you bioidentical hormone replacement therapy, and you're not responding, it could be because your prolactin level is too high.

I also look at IGF-1, which is a mediator of human growth hormone. Last, I look at 25-hydroxy vitamin D, the gold standard measurement to make sure you have enough Vitamin D. I do not look at estrogen or progesterone. I measure that by checking FSH, and LH when necessary.

That's the basic blood work that my patients get, and it's the blood work that I think you need, at least initially, to make sure that you're healthy.

What about breast imaging? I do a full breast exam with my patients, and I teach them how to examine their own breasts. I believe that a woman is more likely to find her own abnormal lumps than imaging studies. In fact, in my patients, that has proven to be true because they're well taught and know what they're looking for. Breast imaging is necessary for women, especially as they're going through menopause, and especially if you decide you're going to use hormone replacement therapy. There are different imaging choices.

One is thermography, which uses heat to sense any inflammation or changes in the blood flow to the breast. It's non-invasive, meaning there are no risk factors to it, but it's not well-accepted in medicine because there are not a lot of providers that read it well.

Mammography is the more accepted option. I almost always order a diagnostic three view mammography, not just a screening test. When I send a patient in for mammography, it's usually because I suspect something's going on with their breast, and I will need three views in order to see what's going on, instead of just a two-view screening. A 3-D mammogram is even better if it's available to my patient. I tell the mammographer what we're looking at, drawing a picture on the order, so they focus on the area of the breast I'm concerned about.

Ultrasound of the breast is also another breast imaging. While breast ultrasound is not accepted for screening, it is used diagnostically. If I have patients who don't want to do mammograms on a regular basis, we use ultrasound with thermography, and mammography only if necessary. According to the patient's imaging results, I may even order an MRI of the breast.

What about bone density? You need a DEXA scan of your hip and spine, at least in the beginning of menopause, and then if you're healthy, every 10 years is fine. If there's any sign of osteopenia, or if you have osteoporosis in your family, you're going to get a DEXA scan more frequently – every 18 months to two years. What I use to look for active bone loss is a urine crosslinks, which measures the proteins that are lost when you're actively reabsorbing your bone because your estrogen levels have fallen. We can recheck urine crosslinks every two to three months once we start treatment like HRT.

After my initial skin evaluation, I recommend an evaluation by a dermatologist if you are at high risk for skin cancer. While I have found skin cancers on my patients, I am not a skin cancer expert, so I send my high-risk patients to a dermatologist for a full skin evaluation. If they're not high-risk, I examine their skin, and teach them what to look for in terms of skin cancer. A lesion that has changed, is very dark in color, or has irregular borders will need to be evaluated.

I ask my patients to get a dental evaluation every year to have their teeth and gums thoroughly examined. The change is a time when you're going to have issues with your gums receding, and any dental work you've had is probably getting a little loose, so you may have some problems with your teeth. The health of your mouth is critical to the health of your heart. Inflammation of your gums can indicate inflammation of your vessels. I've even had patients see their dentist and come back asking for bone density evaluations because of issues picked up on dental X-rays.

Every two years, I recommend an eye exam. Optometrists can do an initial exam and prescribe glasses if necessary. Ophthalmologists are experts on eyes, and perform eye surgery. You need an exam that requires dilating drops in your eyes to make your pupil bigger, so the doctor can look at your macula, or the back of your eye. The back of your eye can show changes related to more than just your vision. Patients have returned from eye exams with requests to check for diabetes, high cholesterol, and other vascular issues because the ophthalmologist saw something concerning during the eye exam. You also need a pressure check for glaucoma. Of course, if you have any issues with your eyes, you're going to have your evaluation sooner than every two years. If needed, I also recommend a hearing evaluation. It may not be needed until you're in your 60's or 70's, and only then if you're having issues with your hearing.

The last screening is a colonoscopy. Around the age of 50, you should have a baseline colonoscopy, and then as recommended upon findings. If everything's healthy, you may not need another one for 10 years. If the gastroenterologist finds any lesions, polyps, or anything suspicious, then you'll need screening more often. If colon cancer runs in your family, you may have a colonoscopy earlier in your 40's.

Personally, I don't do a lot of screening tests for myself. I do my baselines and then I go from there, but I definitely got a colonoscopy at 51 because I had chronic issues with constipation when I was younger, and I wanted to make sure everything was healthy. It was, and I received a 10 year pass.

Effectively partnering with your healthcare provider allows you to ask for what you need.

You have your Menopause Action Plan, so you know what your choices are, and what's happening in your body. If you'd like hormone replacement therapy, you're probably going to need your healthcare provider to prescribe it. If so, you need to partner with them so you can get what you need and then communicate with them effectively once you start using the hormones so that they know how it's working for you.

When counseling with my colleagues – doctors and nurse practitioners who want to learn about hormones – I remind them to communicate with their patients in an open dialogue to allow the woman to explain what's happening with the BHRT they've prescribed. It's a learning experience for both the patient and the healthcare provider.

Being able to communicate what's happening in your body actually helps to teach your healthcare provider more about how the hormones affect you. Don't just assume they know. Healthcare providers have lists of the expected side effects, but not every woman has the same side effects, because every woman is different. Talk frankly with your healthcare provider about what's going on, and about your health goals, and how you can improve your health. They need to know what you're going to do in terms of changing your lifestyle so that you can improve your health and live a strong and vital third book of your life.

Shifting your menopause mindset, educating yourself, getting the support you need to stay accountable to your healing goals, and partnering with your health care provider are all part of the path to empowered menopause. Following this path to empowerment will set you up to receive the gifts of menopause. Your health is key for you to be able to live your best life.

If you're healthy, vital, and hormonally balanced, menopause is going to be a breeze. Postmenopause is truly going to be your golden years, because you're going to have so much joy from living in your truth.

It all starts with finishing your Menopause Action Plan, and partnering with your healthcare provider to get what you need throughout the change, whether you're premenopausal, perimenopausal, menopausal, or postmenopausal.

I'm so excited for you to have started this healing journey, and for you to create your Menopause Action Plan to partner with your healthcare provider.

The change marks your evolution into the woman you were always meant to be. With age, you become even more powerful, because you've learned to accept where you've been, appreciate who you are, and embrace your future. You're finally being your true self.

ACTION ~ Bring your completed Menopause Action Plan to your healthcare provider

Chapter 13

Tools to Thrive

Reading this book is the first step on the journey. Completing your Menopause Action Plan is the second. Bringing your MAP to your health care provider is the third step. Implementing the choices you've made for yourself to thrive in the change is the rest of the journey.

I have tools for you to make your journey easier.

- A fillable Menopause Action Plan - you can download and fill out to bring to your health care provider
- DMAR Nutritional Path to Healing - the same guide I give my patients
- List of Recommended Bloodwork - you can bring to your healthcare provider to order the necessary bloodwork for you
- List of Recommended Screening Tests - you can bring to your healthcare provider to decide together what's necessary for you

Plus, when you sign up to receive these free tools, I'll send you a special MAP discount for Genesis Gold®.

Sign up here for your fillable MAP and free gifts:
GenesisGold.com/MAP

You can find more information on Genesis Gold® here:
GenesisGold.com/GenesisGold

You may find that you need even more help. I have two options for your ongoing support.

Menopause Action Plan Workshop - I created this interactive workshop to help you make the best choices for yourself. In this online group, I cover all the issues you might be up against – like interpreting blood work, menopause weight loss, the best hormone replacement, intimacy issues, and much, much more. As part of the MAP workshop, you get access to an online course, which is updated with my latest recommendations. To access the Menopause Action Plan workshop, go here:

GenesisGold.com/MAP-Workshop/

Hormone Healing Circle - This is the very special group I mentioned in the book where I provide personal health guidance, and help you stay accountable to your healing path. Members have access to all of my most comprehensive online education, covering hormone health, thyroid health, adrenal health, gut health, weight and metabolism, neurological and immune health, and much more. Members also get access to all the research from MAP, every mindset training I've developed, and every tool I've created to help my patients heal. They also get exclusive access to the most compassionate circle of women to help you navigate the change, and more so, become your best self. For more information on our Hormone Healing Circle, go here:

GenesisGold.com/HormoneHealingCircle/

Thank you for including me in your healing journey.

Love and Light,

Deborah

APPENDIX

References

PART 1

Woods, N. F., PhD, RN, & Mitchell, E. S., PhD, RN. (2005) Symptoms during the perimenopause: prevalence, severity, trajectory, and significance in women's lives. The American Journal of Medicine, 118(12):2.

Santoro, N., MD. (2016) Perimenopause: From Research to Practice. Journal of Women's Health, 25(4), 332–339.

Li, S., Holm, K., Gulanick, M., & Lanuza, D. (2000) Perimenopause and the Quality of Lif. Sage Journals, 9(1), 6-23

Perlman, B., Kulak, D., Goldsmith, L. T., Weiss, G. (2018) The etiology of menopause: not just ovarian dysfunction but also a role for the central nervous system. Global Reproductive Health, 3(2), e8.

Dalal, P. K., & Agarwal,, M. (2015) Postmenopausal syndrome. Indian J Psychiatry, 57(2), S222–S232.

Wu, J. M., Zelinski, M. B., Ingram, D. K., & Ottinger, M. A. (2005) Ovarian Aging and Menopause: Current Theories, Hypotheses, and Research Models. Sage Journals, 230(11), 818-828.

PART 2
Common Symptoms

Trudeau, K. J., Ph.D., Ainscough, J. L., B.A., Trant, M., M.S.W., Starker, J., M.S.W., Ph.D., & Cousineau, T., Ph.D. (2011) Identifying the Educational Needs of Menopausal Women: A Feasibility Study. Women's Health Issues, 21(2).

Freedman, R. R., Ph.D. (2014) Menopausal Hot Flashes: Mechanisms, Endocrinology, Treatment. J Steroid Biochem Mol Biol., 142,115–120.

Lee, J., Han, Y., Cho, H. H., & Mee Ran Kim. (2019) Sleep Disorders and Menopause. J Menopausal Med., 25(2), 83–87.

Wesstrom, J., Nilsson, S., Sundstrom-Poromaa, I., & Ulfberg, J. (2008) Restless legs syndrome among women: prevalence, co-morbidity and possible relationship to menopause. Climacteric, 11(5), 422-8

Sieminski, M., Karwacka, M., & Nyka, W. (2012) Restless Legs Syndrome and Hormonal Replacement Therapy in Women at Menopausal Age. Neurology, 78(1)

Lizcano, F., & Guzmán, G. (2014) Estrogen Deficiency and the Origin of Obesity during Menopause Biomed Res Int., 757461

Wharton, W. Ph.D., Gleason, C. E., Ph.D., Olson, S. R. M. S., Carlsson, C. M., M.D., M.S., & Asthana, S., M.D., F.R.C.P. (2012) Neurobiological Underpinnings of the Estrogen – Mood Relationship. Curr Psychiatry, 8(3): 247–256.

Van Wingen, G. A., Van Broekhoven, F., Verkes, R. J., Petersson, K. M., Bäckström, T., Buitelaar, J. K., & Fernández, G. (2008) Progesterone selectively increases amygdala reactivity in women. Molecular Psychiatry, 13, 325–333

Bancroft, J. (2005) The endocrinology of sexual arousal. Journal of Endocrinology, 186(3), 411-427.

Woods, N.F., R.N., Ph.D., Mitchell, E.S., Ph.D., & Julio, K.S., Ph.D., R.N. (2010) Journal of Women's Health, 19(2), 209–218.

Gava,G., Orsili, I., Alvisi, S., Mancini,I., Seracchioli, R., & Meriggiola, M.C. (2019) Cognition, Mood and Sleep in Menopausal Transition: The Role of Menopause Hormone Therapy. Medicina, 55(10), 668.

Not Well Known Symptoms

Freedman, R.R. Ph.D., (2014) Menopausal Hot flashes: Mechanisms, Endocrinology, Treatment. J Steroid Biochem Mol Biol. 142, 115–120.

Lee,J., Han, Y., Cho, H.H., & Kim, M. (2019) Sleep Disorders and Menopause. J Menopausal Med. 25(2), 83–87.

Davis, S.R., Castelo-Branco, C., Chedraui, P., Lumsden, M.A., Nappi, R. E., Shah, D., & Villaseca, P. (2012) Understanding weight gain at menopause. Climacteric, 15(5), 419-29.

Bromberger, J. T., PhD., Kravitz, M. K., DO, MPH. (2011) Mood and Menopause: Findings from the Study of Women's Health Across the Nation (SWAN) over ten years. Obstet Gynecol Clin North Am, 38(3), 609–625.

Leventhal, J. L., MD. (2000) Management of Libido Problems in Menopause. Permanente Journal, 4(3), 29–34.

Woods, N. F., R.N., Ph.D., Mitchell, E. S., Ph.D., & Smith-Di Julio, K., Ph.D., R.N. (2010) Sexual Desire During the Menopausal Transition and Early Postmenopause: Observations from the Seattle Midlife Women's Health Study. J Womens Health (Larchmt), 19(2), 209–218.

Reinberg, S. (2019) Study Links Menopausal Night Sweats to Impaired Thinking. Healthy Day News.

Bryant, C., Judd F. K., Hickey, M. (2012) Anxiety during the menopausal transition: a systematic review. Journal of Affective Disorders, 139(2), 141-8.

Sliwinski, J. R., Johnson, A. K., & Elkins, G. R. (2014) Memory Decline in Peri- and Post-menopausal Women: The Potential of Mind–Body Medicine to Improve Cognitive Performance. Integrative Medicine Insights, 9, 17–23.

Scheyer, O., Rahman, A., Hristov, H., Berkowitz, C., Isaacson, R.S., Diaz Brinton, R., & Mosconi, L. (2018) Female Sex and Alzheimer's Risk: The Menopause Connection. *The Journal of Prevention of Alzheimer's Disease*, 5(4), 225–230.

American Academy of Neurology (2009) Menopause Transition May Cause Trouble Learning. Science Daily.

Nicol-Smith, L. (1996) Causality, menopause, and depression: a critical review of literature. BMJ, 313, 1229-1232.

Cohen, L. S., MD, Soares, C. N., MD, PhD, & Vitonis, A. F., BA. (2006) Risk for New Onset of Depression During the Menopausal Transition. Arch Gen Psychiatry, 63(4), 385-390, 223-225.

Smoller, J. W., MD, ScD, Pollack, M.H., MD, & Wassertheil-Smoller, S., PhD. (2003) Prevalence and Correlates of Panic Attacks in Postmenopausal Women. Arch Intern Med, 163(17), 2041-2050.

Sammaritano, L. R. (2012) Menopause in patients with autoimmune diseases. Autoimmunity Review, 11(6–7), A430-A436.

Shah, S. (2012) Hormonal Link to Autoimmune Allergies. ISRN Allergy, 2012, 910437.

Perry, S. (2021) Menopause and allergies: how to breathe easy. Gennev.

Stenberg, A. G., & Ulmsten, H. U. (1995) The prevalence of urogenital symptoms in postmenopausal women. Maturitas, 22(1), S17-S20.

Pace, F., Watnick, P.I. (2020) The Interplay of Sex Steroids, the Immune Response, and the Intestinal Microbiota. Trends in Microbiology.

Digestive Tract Responses to the Change:

Mayneris-Perxachs, J., Arnoriaga-Rodríguez, M., Luque-Córdoba, D., Priego-Capote, F., Pérez-Brocal, V., Moya, A., Burokas, A., Maldonado, R., & Fernández-Real, J.M. (2020) Gut microbiota steroid sexual dimorphism and its impact on gonadal steroids: influences of obesity and menopausal status. Microbiome, 8, 136.

Black, H. E. (1988) The effects of steroids upon the gastrointestinal tract. Toxicol Pathol, 16(2), 213-22.

Amure, B. o., & Omole, A. A. (1970) Sex hormones and acid gastric secretion induced with carbachol, histamine, and gastrin. Gut. 11, 641-645.

Keshavarzi, Z., Zahedi, M. J., & Haddad, M. K. (2011) The Effects of Female Sex Steroids on Gastric Secretory Responses of Rat Following Traumatic Brain Injury. Iranian Journal of Basic Medical Sciences, 14(3), 231-239.

Triadafilopoulos, G., Finlayson, M., & Grellet, C. (1998) Bowel dysfunction in postmenopausal women. Women Health. 27(4), 55-66.

Heitkemper, M. M., PhD. & Lin Chang, L., MD. (2009) Do Fluctuations in Ovarian Hormones Affect Gastrointestinal Symptoms in Women With Irritable Bowel Syndrome? Gender Medicine, 6(2), 152–167.

Messa, C., Maselli, M. A., Cavallini, A., Caruso, M. L., Pezzolla, F., & Leo, A Di. (1990) Sex steroid hormone receptors and human gallbladder motility in vitro. Digestion, 46(4),214-9.

Dornschneider, G., Izbicki, J. R., Wilker, D. K., & Schweiberer, L. (1990) The effects of sex steroids on colon carcinogenesis. Anti-cancer Drugs, 1(1),15-21.

Hutson, W. R., Roehrkasse, R. L., & Wald, A. (1989) Influence of gender and menopause on gastric emptying and motility. Gastroenterology, 96(1), 11-17

Dermatological and Connective Tissue Responses to the Change:

Mac Bride, M. B., MBBCh, Rhodes, D. J., MD, & Shuster, L. T., MD. (2010) Vulvovaginal Atrophy. Mayo Clinic Proceedings, 85(1), 87–94.

Bhardwaj, A., & Bhardwaj, S. V. (2012) Effect of menopause on women's periodontium. Journal of Mid-Life Health, 3(1), 5–9.

Nair, P. A. (2014) Dermatosis associated with menopause. Journal of Mid-Life Health, 5(4),168–175.

Duarte, G. V., MD, PhD, Moura Trigo, A. C., MD, De Fátima Paim de Oliveira, M., PhD. (2016) Skin Disorders During Menopause. Cutis, 97(2), E16-E23.

Reus, T. L., Carla AbdoBrohem, C., Schuck, D. C., & Lorencini, M. (2020) Revisiting the effects of menopause on the skin: Functional changes, clinical studies, in vitro models and therapeutic alternatives. Mechanisms of Ageing and Development, 185, 111193.

El Safoury, O., Rashid, L., & Ibrahim, M. (2010) A Study of Androgen and Estrogen Receptors α, β in Skin Tags. Indian Journal of Dermatology, 55(1), 20–24.

Pariath, K., & Nair, P. A. (2019) A Cross-Sectional Study on the Dermatoses in Postmenopausal Patients at a Rural-Based Tertiary Health Care Center. Indian Journal of Dermatology, 64(5), 360–365.

Mirmirani, P. (2011) Hormonal changes in menopause: do they contribute to a 'midlife hair crisis' in women? Br J Dermatol., 165(3), 7-11.

Trutnovsky, G., Guzman Rojas, R., Mann, K. P., & Dietz, H. P. (2014) Urinary incontinence: the role of menopause. Menopause, 21(4), 399-402.

Thulkar, J., & Singh, S. (2015) Overview of research studies on osteoporosis in menopausal women since the last decade. Journal of Mid-Life Health, 6(3), 104–107.

Feola, A. J., Sherwood, J. M., Pardue, M. T., Overby, D. R., & Ethier, C. R. (2020) Age and Menopause Effects on Ocular Compliance and Aqueous Outflow. Investigative Ophthalmology & Visual Science, 61, 16.

Nervous System Responses to the Change:

Ripa, P., Ornello, R., Degan, D., Tiseo, C., Stewart, J., Pistoia, F., Carolei, A., & Sacco, S. (2015) Migraine in menopausal women: a systematic review. International Journal of Women's Health, 7, 773–782.

Vaidya, R. (2012) Burning mouth syndrome at menopause: Elusive etiology. Journal of Mid-Life Health, 3(1), 3–4.

Magliano, M. (2010) Menopausal arthralgia: Fact or fiction. Maturitas. 67(1), 29-33.

Khadilkar, S. S. (2019) Musculoskeletal Disorders and Menopause. The Journal of Obstetrics and Gynecology of India, 69, 99–103.

Craft, R. M. (2007) Modulation of pain by estrogens. Pain, 132(1), S3-S12.

Crandall, C. J., MD, MS, Markovic, D., MS, Huang, M., DrPH, &. Greendale, G. A., MD. (2010) Predictors of Breast Discomfort among Women Initiating Menopausal Hormone Therapy. Menopause, 17(3), 462–470.

Mutneja, P., Dhawan, P., Raina, A., & Sharma, G. (2012) Menopause and the oral cavity. Indian Journal of Endocrinology and Metabolism, 16(4), 548–551.

University of Jyväskylä. (2017) Menopause and estrogen affect muscle function. ScienceDaily.

Singh, A., Asif, N., Singh, P. N., & Hossain, M. M. (2016) Motor Nerve Conduction Velocity In Postmenopausal Women with Peripheral Neuropathy. Journal of Clinical & Diagnostic Research, 10(12), CC13–CC16.

Lee, J. O., Kang, S. G., Kim, S. H., Park, S. J., & Song, S. W. (2011) The Relationship between Menopausal Symptoms and Heart Rate Variability in Middle Aged Women. Korean Journal of Family Medicine, 32(5): 299–305.

Ogun, O. A., MD, Büki, B., MD, PhD, Cohn, E. S., MD, Janky, K. L., AuD, PhD, & Lundberg, Y. W., PhD. (2014) Menopause and benign paroxysmal positional vertigo. Menopause, 21(8), 886-889.

Caruso, S., Grillo, C., Agnello, C., Di Mari, L., Farina, M., & Serra, A. (2004) Olfactometric and rhinomanometric outcomes in postmenopausal women treated with hormone therapy: a prospective study. Human Reproduction, 19(12), 2959-2964.

Tarumi, W., & Shinohara, K. (2020) Women's body odour during the ovulatory phase modulates testosterone and cortisol levels in men. PLoS One, 15(3), e0230838.

Rantala, M. J., Peter Eriksson, C. J., Vainikka, A., & Kortet, R. (2006) Male steroid hormones and female preference for male body odor. Evolution and Human Behavior, 27(4), 259-269.

Risk Factors:

Preidt, R. (2015) Chronic Fatigue Syndrome Linked to Early Menopause. HealthyDay News.

Lenart-Lipińska, M., Matyjaszek-Matuszek, B., Woźniakowska, E., Janusz Solski, J., Tarach, J. S., & Paszkowski, T. (2014) Polycystic ovary syndrome: clinical implication in perimenopause. Przegland Menopauzalny, 13(6), 348-351.

Sekhar, S. T.V.D., Medarametla, S., Rahman, A., & Adapa, S. S. (2015) Early Menopause in Type 2 Diabetes – A Study from a South Indian Tertiary Care Centre. Journal of Clinical & Diagnostic Research, 9(10), OC08-OC10.

Kim, C. (2012) Does menopause increase diabetes risk? Strategies for diabetes prevention in midlife women. Women's Health, 8(2), 155-67.

Helfenstein Fonseca, M. I., Tande da Silva, I., & G Ferreira, S. R. (2017) Impact of menopause and diabetes on atherogenic lipid profile: is it worth to analyse lipoprotein subfractions to assess cardiovascular risk in women? Diabetology & Metabolic Syndrome, 9,22.

Shufelt, C., Dutra, E., Torbati, T., & Ramineni, T. (2019) A clinical prescription for heart health in midlife women. Maturitas, 119, 46-53.

Sievert, L. L., Waddle, D., Canali, K. (2001) Marital status and age at natural menopause: considering pheromonal influence. American journal of Human Biology: the official journal of the Human Biology Council, 13(4), 479-85.

Vaughn Fielder, K., & Robinson Kurpius, S. E. Marriage, Stress and Menopause: Midlife Challenges and Joys. Counseling Psychology Program, 19(1-2), 5.

Langton, C. R., MSW, MPH, Whitcomb, B. W., PhD., Purdue-Smithe, A. C., PhD., Sievert, L. L., PhD., Hankinson, S. E., ScD., Manson, J. E., MD, DrPH., Rosner, B. A., PhD., & Bertone-Johnson, E. R., ScD. (2020) Association of Parity and Breastfeeding With Risk of Early Natural Menopause. JAMA Network Open, 3(1), e1919615.

Aloia, J. F., Cohn, S. H., Vaswani, A., Yeh, J. K., Yuen, K., & Ellis, K. (1985) Risk factors for postmenopausal osteoporosis. The American Journal of Medicine, 78(1), 95-100.

McCarthy, M., & Raval, A. P. (2020) The peri-menopause in a woman's life: a systemic inflammatory phase that enables later neurodegenerative disease. Journal of Neuroinflammation, 17, 317.

Increased Alzheimer's Risk During Menopause Transition. (2019) Cure Alzheimer's Fund.

Devere, R., MD, FAAN. (2019) Dementia Insights: Cognitive Consequences of Perimenopause. Practical Neurology.

Tang, J. Y., Spaunhurst, K. M., Chlebowski, R. T., Wactawski-Wende, J., Keiser, E., Thomas, F., Anderson, M. L., Zeitouni, N. C., Larson, J. C., & Stefanick, M. L. (2011) Menopausal hormone therapy and risks of melanoma and nonmelanoma skin cancers: women's health initiative randomized trials. Journal of the National Cancer Institute, 103(19), 1469-1475.

Aruna Surakasula, A., Nagarjunapu, G. C., & Raghavaiah, K. V. (2014) A comparative study of pre- and post-menopausal breast cancer: Risk factors, presentation, characteristics and management. Journal of Research in Pharmacy Practice, 3(1), 12–18.

Johnson, J. R., Lacey Jr., J. V., Lazovich, D., Geller, M. A., Schairer, C., Schatzkin, A., & Flood, A. (2009) Menopausal Hormone Therapy and Risk of Colorectal Cancer. Cancer Epidemiology, Biomarkers & Prevention, 18(1), 196.

Eshtiaghi, R., Esteghamati, A., & Nakhjavani, M. (2009) Menopause is an independent predictor of Metabolic syndrome in Iranian women. Maturitas, 65(3):262-266

Carr, M.C. (2003) The Emergence of the Metabolic Syndrome with Menopause. The Journal of Clinical Endocrinology & Metabolism, 88(6), 2404–2411.

PART 3

Hypothalamus Connections

Warrier Mitra, S., Hoskin, E., Yudkovitz, J., Pear, L., Wilkinson, H. A., Hayashi, S., Pfaff, D. W., Ogawa, S., Rohrer, S. P., Schaeffer, J. M., Mcewen, B. S., & Alves, S. E. (2003) Immunolocalization of Estrogen Receptor in the Mouse Brain: Comparison with Estrogen Receptor. Endocrinology, 144(5), 2055-2067.

White, M. M., Sheffer, I., Teeter, J., & Apostolakis, E. M. (2007) Hypothalamic progesterone receptor-A mediates gonadotropin surges, self priming and receptivity in estrogen-primed female mice. Journal of Molecular Endocrinology, 38(1-2), 35-50.

Lloyd, J. M., Scarbrough, K., Weiland, N. G., & Wise, P. M. (1991) Age-related changes in proopiomelanocortin (POMC) gene expression in the periarcuate region of ovariectomized rats. Endocrinology, 129(4), 1896-1902

Ferguson, A. V., Latchford, K. J., & Samson, W. K. (2009) The Paraventricular Nucleus of the Hypothalamus A Potential Target for Integrative Treatment of Autonomic Dysfunction. Expert Opin Ther Targets, 12(6), 717–727.

Diaz Brinton, R., Thompson, R. F., Foy, M. R., Baudry, M., Wang, J., Finch, C. E., Morgan, T. E., Stanczyk, F. Z., Pike, C. J., & Nilsen, J. (2008) Progesterone Receptors: Form and Function in Brain. Front Neuroendocrinol, 29(2), 313–339.

Rybaczyk, L. A., Bashaw, M. J., Pathak, D. R., Moody, S. M., Gilders, R. M., & Holzschu, D. L. (2005) An overlooked connection: serotonergic mediation of estrogen-related physiology and pathology. BMC Womens Health, 5, 12.

Celec, P., Ostatníková, D., Hodosy, J. (2015) On the effects of testosterone on brain behavioral functions. Frontiers in Neuroscience.

Placzek, K., MD. (2018) The Impact of Hormones on Serotonin in Depression. The ZRT Laboratory Blog.

Newhouse, P., M.D. & Dumas, J., Ph.D. (2015) Estrogen-Cholinergic Interactions: Implications for Cognitive Aging. Hormones and behavior. Hormones and Behavior, 173–185.

Lee, J., Han, Y., Cho, H. H., & Kim, M. (2019) Sleep Disorders and Menopause. Journal of Menopausal Medicine, 25(2), 83–87.

Ghosh, M., Rodriguez-Garcia, M., & Wira, C. R. (2014) The Immune System in Menopause: Pros and Cons of Hormone Therapy. The Journal of Steroid Biochemistry and Molecular Biology, 0, 171–175.

Rajagopalan, A., Jinu, K. V., Sailesh, K. S., Mishra, S., Reddy, U. K., & Mukkadan, J. K. (2017) Understanding the links between vestibular and limbic systems regulating emotions. Journal of Natural Science, Biology and Medicine, 8(1), 11–15.

Nishida, M., Miyagawa, J. I., Tokunaga, K., Yamamoto, K., Keno, Y., Kobatake, T., Yoshida, S., Nakamura, T., Odaka, H., Ikeda, H., Hanafusa, T., Yamashita, S., Kameda-Takemura, S., & Matsuzawa, Y. (1997) Early morphologic changes of atherosclerosis induced by ventromedial hypothalamic lesion in the spontaneously diabetic Goto-Kakizaki rat. The Journal of Laboratory and Clinical Medicine, 129(2):200-7.

Khomulo, P. S., Dmitrieva, N. A., & Eliner, G. I. (1976) Atherosclerosis in rabbits induced by prolonged electrical stimulation of the hypothalamus. Biull Eksp Biol Med, 82(11), 1294-1296.

Guijarro, A., Laviano, A., & Meguid, M. M. (2006) Hypothalamic integration of immune function and metabolism. Progress in Brain Research, 153, 367-405.

Bellavance, M. & Rivest, S. (2014) The HPA – immune axis and the immunomodulatory actions of glucocorticoids in the brain. Frontiers in Immunology.

Kiess, W., & Belohradsky, B. H. (1986) Endocrine regulation of the immune system. Klinische Wochenschrift, 64, 1–7.

Overlie, I., Mørkrid, L., Andersson, A., Skakkebaek, N. E., Moen, M. H., & Holte, A. (2005) Inhibin A and B as markers of menopause: a five-year prospective longitudinal study of hormonal changes during the menopausal transition. Acta Obstet Gynecol Scand, 84(3), 281-5.

PART 5

Hormone Replacement Therapy

Thompson, J. J., Ritenbaugh, C., & Nichter, M. (2017) Why women choose compounded bioidentical hormone therapy: lessons from a qualitative study of menopausal decision-making. BMC Women's Health, 17(1), 97.

Çilgin, H. (2019) Predictors of Initiating Hormone Replacement Therapy in Postmenopausal Women: A Cross-Sectional Study. The Scientific World Journal, 2019, 1814804.

Iftikhar, S., Shuster, L. T., Johnson, R. E., Jenkins, S. J., & Wahner-Roedler, D. L. (2011) Use of bioidentical compounded hormones for menopausal concerns: cross-sectional survey in an academic menopause center. Journal of Women's Health, 20(4), 559-65.

Beaber, E. F., Buist, D. S. M., Barlow, W. E., Malone, K. E., Reed, S. D., & Li, C. I. (2014) Recent Oral Contraceptive Use by Formulation and Breast Cancer Risk among Women 20 to 49 Years of Age. Cancer Research, 74(15), 4078-4089.

Stute, P., Wildt, L., & Neulen, J. (2018) The impact of micronized progesterone on breast cancer risk: a systematic review. Climacteric. 21(2), 111-122.

Lobo, R. A. (2013) Where Are We 10 Years After the Women's Health Initiative? The Journal of Clinical Endocrinology & Metabolism, 98(5), 1771–1780.

Beral, V., Peto, R., Pirie, K., & Reeves, G. (2019) Type and timing of menopausal hormone therapy and breast cancer risk: individual participant meta-analysis of the worldwide epidemiological evidence. The Lancet, 394 (10204), 1159-1168.

Gallagher, J. C., MD. & Tella, S. H, MD. (2014) Prevention and treatment of postmenopausal osteoporosis. The Journal of Steroid Biochemistry and Molecular Biology, 142, 155–170.

Del Ghianda, S., Tonacchera, M., & Vitti, P. (2014) Thyroid and Menopause. Climacteric, 17(3), 225-234.

Fanciulli, G., Delitala, A., & Delitala, G. (2009) Growth hormone, menopause and ageing: no definite evidence for 'rejuvenation' with growth hormone. Human Reproduction Update, 15(3), 341–358.

Panjari, M., & Davis, S. R. (2007) DHEA therapy for women: effect on sexual function and wellbeing. Human Reproduction Update, 13(3), 239–248.

Meldrum, D. R., Defazio, J. D., Erlik Y., Lu, J. K., Wolfsen, A. F., Carlson, H. E., Hershman, J. M., & Judd, H. L. (1984) Pituitary hormones during the menopausal hot flash. Obstet Gynecol, 64(6), 752-756.

Guthrie, J. R., Dennerstein, L., Hopper, J. L., & Burger, H. G. (1996) Hot flushes, menstrual status, and hormone levels in a population-based sample of midlife women. Obstet Gynecol, 88(3), 437-442.

Overlie, I., Moen, M. H., Holte, A., & Finset, A. (2002) Androgens and estrogens in relation to hot flushes during the menopausal transition. Maturitas, 41(1), 69-77.

Prior, J. C. (2018) Progesterone for treatment of symptomatic menopausal women. Climacteric, 21(4), 358-365.

Lieberman, A., & Curtis, L. (2017) In Defense of Progesterone: A Review of the Literature. Alternative Therapies in Health and Medicine, 23(6), 24-32.

Monaco, K., & Writer, S. (2020) Hormone Levels Tied to Future Breast Cancer Risk. MedPage Today, 86155.

Bethesda, MD. (1998) The p53 tumor suppressor protein. National Center for Biotechnology Information. Genes and Disease, NBK22268.

Bu, S. Z., Yin, D. L., Ren, X. H., Jiang, L. Z., Wu, Z. J., Gao, Q. R., & Pei, G. (1997) Progesterone induces apoptosis and up-regulation of p53 expression in human ovarian carcinoma cell lines. Cancer, 79(10), 1944-50.

Dunphy, K. A., Blackburn, A. C., Yan, H., O'Connell, L. R., & Jerry, D. J. (2008) Estrogen and progesterone induce persistent increases in p53-dependent apoptosis and suppress mammary tumors in BALB/c-Trp53+/-mice. Breast Cancer Research, 10, R43.

Azeez, J., Sithul, H., Hariharan, I., Sreekumar, S., Prabhakar, J., Sreeja, S., & Pillai, M. (2015) Progesterone regulates the proliferation of breast cancer cells – in vitro evidence. Dovepress, 2015(9), 5987 —5999.

Tamimi, R. M., ScD., Hankinson, S. E., ScD., Chen, W. Y., MD, Rosner, B., PhD., Colditz, G. A., MD., DrPH. Combined Estrogen and Testosterone Use and Risk of Breast Cancer in Postmenopausal Women. Arch Intern Med, 166(14), 1483-1489.

Glaser, R. L., York, A. E., & Dimitrakakis, C. (2019) Incidence of invasive breast cancer in women treated with testosterone implants: a prospective 10-year cohort study. BMR Cancer, 19, 1271.

Jehan, S., Jean-Louis, G., Zizi, F., Auguste, E., Pandi-Perumal, S. R., Gupta, R., Attarian, H., McFarlane, S. I., Hardeland, R., & Brzezinski, A. (2017) Sleep, Melatonin, and the Menopausal Transition: What Are the Links? Sleep Science, 10(1), 11-18.

Parandavar, N., Abdali, K., Keshtgar, S., Emamghoreishi, M., & Amooee, S. (2014) The Effect of Melatonin on Climacteric Symptoms in Menopausal Women; A Double-Blind, Randomized

Controlled, Clinical Trial. Iranian Journal of Public Health, 43(10), 1405–1416.

Kripke, D. F., Kline, L. E., Shadan, F. F., Dawson, A., Poceta, J. S., & Elliott, J. A. (2006) Melatonin effects on luteinizing hormone in postmenopausal women: a pilot clinical trial NCT00288262. BMC Women's Health, 6, 8.

Scheffers, C. S., Armstrong, S., Cantineau, AEP., Farquhar, C., & Jordan, V. (2015) Dehydroepiandrosterone for women in the peri- or postmenopausal phase. Cochrane Database of Systematic Reviews, 1, CD011066.

Tribble, D. L., Glover, M. R., & Lambeth, J. D. (1987) Pregnenolone production by adrenal mitochondria: a new high-performance liquid chromatographic analytical method for cholesterol side-chain cleavage. Journal of Chromatography, 414(2), 411-6.

Fluker, M. R., MD, FRCSC. (2001) HRT in older Women: Is it ever too late? BC Medical Journal, 43(9), 517-521.

Lotta Järvstråt, L., Spetz Holm, AC. E., Lindh-Åstrand, L., Hoffmann, M. J., Fredrikson, M. G., & Hammar, M. L. (2015) Use of hormone therapy in Swedish women aged 80 years or older. Menopause, 22(3), 275-278.

Clanton, M. A. Menopause: Understanding and Managing the transition using essential oils vs. traditional allopathic medicine. Australasian College of Health Sciences.

Alternative Therapies

Mayo, J. L., MD., FACOG. (1998) Black Cohosh and Chasteberry: Herbs Valued by Women for Centuries. Clinical Nutrition Insights, 6, 15.

Leea, M. S., Shinb, BC., Yanga, E. J., Limc, HJ., & Ernst, E. (2011) Maca (Lepidium meyenii) for treatment of menopausal symptoms: A systematic review. Maturitas, 70, 227-233.

Brooks, N. A., BSci (Hons), Wilcox, G., BMedSc (Hons), MD, FRACP, FRCPA, Walker, K. Z., MND, PhD, Ashton, J. F., MSc, PhD, Cox, M. B., MSPH, PhD, & Stojanovska, L., MSc, PhD. (2008) Beneficial effects of Lepidium meyenii (Maca) on psychological symptoms and measures of sexual dysfunction in postmenopausal women are not related to estrogen or androgen content. Menopause: The Journal of The North American Menopause Society, 15(6), 1157-1162.

Geller, S. E., Ph.D., & Studee, L., MPH. (2005) Botanical and Dietary Supplements for Menopausal Symptoms: What Works, What Doesn't. Journal of Women's Health, 14(7), 634–649.

Villines, Z. (2020) Essential oils and menopause: Can they help?. MedicalNewsToday, 317918.

Milart, P., Woźniakowska, E., & Wrona, W. (2018) Selected vitamins and quality of life in menopausal women. Prz Menopauzalny, 17(4), 175–179.

Dennehy, C., & Tsourounis, C. (2010) A review of select vitamins and minerals used by postmenopausal women. Maturitas, 66(4), 370-80.

Price, C. T., Langford, J. R., & Liporace, F. A. (2012) Essential Nutrients for Bone Health and a Review of their Availability in the Average North American Diet. Open Orthop J., 6, 143–149.

Schwalfenberg, G. K. (2017) Vitamins K1 and K2: The Emerging Group of Vitamins Required for Human Health. Journal of Nutrition and Metabolism, 2017, 6254836.

Hamidi, M. S., Gajic-Veljanoski, O., & Cheung, A. M. (2013) Vitamin K and bone health. J Clin Densitom, 16(4), 409-13.

Price, C. T., Koval, K. J., & Langford, J. R. (2013) International Journal of Endocrinology, 2013, 216783.

Jugdaohsingh, R. (2009) Silicon and bone health. J Nutr Health Aging, 11(2), 99-110.

Fogelman, I., & Blake, G. M. (2005) Strontium ranelate for the treatment of osteoporosis. BMJ, 330(7505), 1400-1401.

Vannucci, L., Fossi, C., Quattrini, S., Guasti, L., Pampaloni, B., Grochi, G., Giusti, F., Romagnoli, C., Cianferotti, Marcucci, G., & Brandi, M. L. (2018) Calcium Intake in Bone Health: A Focus on Calcium-Rich Mineral Waters. Nutrients, 10(12), 1930.

(2018) National Osteoporosis Foundation, A Guide to Calcium-Rich Food.

Malde, M. K., Bugel, S., Kristensen, M., Malde, K., Graff, I. E., and Pedersen, J. I. (2010) Calcium from salmon and cod bone is well absorbed in young healthy men: a double-blinded randomised crossover design. Nutrition and Metabolism, 7, 61.

Dalessandri, K. M., Firestone, G. L., Fitch, M. D., Bradlow, H. L., & Bjeldanes, L. F. (2004) Pilot study: effect of 3,3'-diindolylmethane supplements on urinary hormone metabolites in postmenopausal women with a history of early-stage breast cancer. Nutrition and Cancer, 50(2),161-167.

Kim, JM., & Park, Y. J. (2017) Probiotics in the Prevention and Treatment of Postmenopausal Vaginal Infections: Review Article. Journal of Menopausal Medicine, 23(3), 139-145.

Secades, J. J., & Frontera, G. (1995) CDP-choline: pharmacological and clinical review. Methods Find Exp Clin Pharmacol, 17(B), 1-54.

Wu, W. H., Lu, S. C., Wang, T. F., Jou, H. J., & Wang, T. A. (2005) Effects of docosahexaenoic acid supplementation on blood lipids, estrogen metabolism, and in vivo oxidative stress in postmenopausal vegetarian women. European Journal of Clinical Nutrition, 60, 386–392

Cao, W., Ma, Z., Rasenick, M. M., Yeh, S., & Yu, J. (2012) N-3 polyunsaturated fatty acids shift estrogen signaling to inhibit human breast cancer cell growth. PLoS One, 7(12), e52838.

Choi, JE., & Park, Y. (2017) EPA and DHA, but not ALA, have antidepressant effects with 17β-estradiol injection via regulation of a neurobiological system in ovariectomized rats. The Journal of Nutritional Biochemistry, 49, 101-109.

Johnson, A., PhD, Roberts, L., & Elkins, G., PhD. (2019) Complementary and Alternative Medicine for Menopause. Journal of Evidenced-Based Integrative Medicine, 24, 2515690X19829380.

Part 5

Lifestyle Recommendations

Soleymani, M., Siassi, F., Qorbani, M., Khosravi, S., Aslany, Z., Abshirini, M., Zolfaghari, G., & Sotoudeh, G. (2019) Dietary patterns and their association with menopausal symptoms: a cross-sectional study. Menopause, 26(4), 365-372.

Abshirini, M., Siassi, F., Koohdani, F., Qorbani, M., Khosravi, S., Hedayati, M., Aslani, Z., Soleymani, M., & Sotoudeh, G. (2018) Dietary total antioxidant capacity is inversely related to menopausal symptoms: a cross-sectional study among Iranian postmenopausal women. Nutrition, 55-56:161-167.

Pugliese, G., Dr, Barrea, L., Dr, Laudisio, D., Dr, Aprano, S., Dr, Castellucci, B., Dr, Framondi, L., Dr, Di Matteo, R., Dr, Savastano, S. Prof, Colao, A., Prof, & Muscogiuri, G., Dr. (2020) Mediterranean diet as tool to manage obesity in menopause: A narrative review. Nutrition, 79-80:110991.

Register, T. C., Ph.D., Cline, J. M., D.V.M., Ph.D., & Shively, C. A., Ph.D. (2003) Health Issues in Postmenopausal Women Who Drink. National Institute on Alcohol Abuse and Alcoholism.

Barclay, L., MD. (2014) Caffeine May Worsen Vasomotor Symptoms of Menopause. Medscape.

Lee, O. J., Kangm, S. G., Kim, S. H., Park, S. J., & Song, S. W. (2011) The Relationship between Menopausal Symptoms and Heart Rate Variability in Middle Aged Women. Korean Journal of Family Medicine, 32(5), 299–305.

Harvey, P. J., BMBS, PhD, FRACP, O'Donnell, E. PhD, Picton, P., MASc, MA, Morris, B. L. RN, Notarius, C. F. PhD, Floras, J. S. MD, DPhil, FRCPC. (2016) After-exercise heart rate variability is attenuated in postmenopausal women and unaffected by estrogen therapy. Menopause, 23(4), 390-395.

Tulppo, M. P., Mäkikallio, T. H., Seppänen, T., Laukkanen, R., & Huikuri, H. V. (1998) Vagal modulation of heart rate during exercise: effects of age and physical fitness. Am J Physiol, 274(2), H424-429.

Lin, YY., & Lee, SD. (2018) Cardiovascular Benefits of Exercise Training in Postmenopausal Hypertension. Int J Mol Sci, 19(9), 2523.

Mishra, N., Mishra, V. N., & Devanshi. (2011) Exercise beyond menopause: Dos and Don'ts. J Midlife Health, 2(2), 51-56.

Grove K. A., & Londeree B. R. (1992) Bone density in postmenopausal women: high impact vs low impact exercise. *Med Sci Sports Exerc.* 24, 1190–1194.

Muffet, J. K., Torgenson, D., Bell-Syer, S., Jackson, D., Llewlyn-Phill-lips, H., Farrin, A., & Barber, J. (1999) Randomized controlled trial of exercise for low back pain: clinical outcomes, costs and preferences. Br Med J., 3, 279–83.

Aleari, C. A. (1999) A randomized trial of a combined physical activity and environmental intervention in nursing home residents: Do sleep and agitation improve. J Am Gerontol Soc., 47, 784–791.

Daley, A., Stokes-Lampard, H., & MacArthur, C. (2011) Exercise for vasomotor menopausal symptoms. Cochrane Database Syst Rev., 5, CD006108.

Shah, R. (2009) Approaches to the prevention of bone health throughout life, Target Osteoporosis. IMS insight, 3, 39–46.

Bonaiuti, D., Cranney, A., Lovine, R., Kemper, HH., Negrini, S., Robinson, V., Kemper, H. C., Wells, G., Tugwell, P., & Cranney, A. (2002) Exercise for preventing and treating osteoporosis in postmenopausal women. Cochrane Database Syst Rev., 2, CD000333.

Bailey, T. G., Mielke, G. I., Skinner, T. S., Anderson, D., Porter-Steele, J., Balaam, S., Young, L., & McCarthy, A. L. (2020) Physical activity and menopausal symptoms in women who have received menopause-inducing cancer treatments: results from the Women's Wellness After Cancer Program. Menopause, 28(2), 142-149.

Dąbrowska, J., Dąbrowska-Galas, M., Rutkowska, M., & Michalski, B. A. (2016) Twelve-week exercise training and the quality of life in menopausal women – clinical trial. Prz Menopauzalny, 15(1), 20–25.

Wong, C., Hon-Kei Yip, B., Gao, T., Yuk Lam, K. Y., Sum Woo, D. M., King Yip, A. L., Yu Chin, C., Yin Tang, W. P., Tse Choy, M. M., Key Tsang, K. W., Ho, S. C., Wah Ma, H. S., & Shan Wong, S. Y. (2018) Mindfulness-Based Stress Reduction (MBSR) or Psychoeducation for the Reduction of Menopausal Symptoms: A Randomized, Controlled Clinical Trial. Sci Rep., 8, 6609.

Morrison, L. A., PhD, Sievert, L. L., PhD, Brown, D. E., PhD, Rahberg, N., BA, and Reza, A., BA. (2010) Relationships between menstrual and menopausal attitudes and associated demographic and health characteristics: The Hilo Women's Health Study. Women Health, 50(5), 397–413.

Ayers, B., Forshaw, M., & Hunter, M. S. (2010) The impact of attitudes towards the menopause on women's symptom experience: A systematic review. Maturitas, 65(1), 28-36.

Bromberger, J. T., PhD & Kravitz, H. M., DO, MPH. Mood and Menopause: Findings from the Study of Women's Health Across the Nation (SWAN) over ten years. Obstet Gynecol Clin North Am., 38(3), 609–625.

Erbil, N. (2018) Attitudes towards menopause and depression, body image of women during menopause. Alexandria Journal of Medicine, 54(3), 241-246.

Rance, N. E. (2009) Menopause and the Human Hypothalamus: Evidence for the Role of Kisspeptin/Neurokinin B Neurons in the Regulation of Estrogen Negative Feedback. Peptides, 30(1), 111-122.

Empowered Menopause

Walter, F. M., Emery, J. D., Rogers, M., & Britten, N. Women's views of optimal risk communication and decision making in general practice consultations about the menopause and hormone replacement therapy. Patient Educ Couns., 53(2), 121-8.

Parish, S. J., Nappi, R. E., & Kingsberg, S. (2018) Perspectives on counseling patients about menopausal hormone therapy: strategies in a complex data environment Menopause, 25(8), 937-949.

Portman, D. J., Gass, M. L. S. Vulvovaginal Atrophy Terminology Consensus Conference Panel. Genitourinary Syndrome of Menopause: New Terminology for Vulvovaginal Atrophy from the International Society for the Study of Women's Sexual Health and

The North American Menopause Society. J Sex Med, 11(12), 2865-2872.

Peng, W., MMed, Adams, J., PhD, Sibbritt, D. W., PhD., Frawley, J. E., MClinSci. (2014) Critical review of complementary and alternative medicine use in menopause focus on prevalence, motivation, decision-making, and communication. Menopause, 21 (5), 536-548.

Buchanan, M. C., Villagran, M. M. & Ragan, S. L. (2009) Women, Menopause, and (Ms.)Information: Communication About the Climacteric. Health Communication, 14(1).

Walter, F. M., Emery, J. D., Rogers, M., & Britten, N. (2014) Women's views of optimal risk communication and decision making in general practice consultations about the menopause and hormone replacement therapy. Patient Educ Couns, 53(2), 121-8.

Yazdkhasti, M., Simbar, M., & Abdi, F. (2015) Empowerment and Coping Strategies in Menopause Women: A Review. Iran Red Crescent Med J., 17(3), e18944.

Yazdkhasti, M., Negarandeh, R., & Moghadam, Z. B. An empowerment model of Iranian women for the management of menopause: a grounded theory study. Int J Qual Stud Health Well-being. 2019; 14(1): 1665958.

Yazdkhasti, M., Simbar, M., & Abdi, F. (2015) Empowerment and Coping Strategies in Menopause Women: A Review Iranian Red Crescent Medical Journal, 17(3).

Nickel, W. K., MPH, Weinberger, S. E., MD, Guze, P. A., MD, MS. (2018) Principles for Patient and Family Partnership in Care: An American College of Physicians Position Paper. Annals of Internal Medicine.

About the Author

Deborah Maragopoulos FNP graduated from UCLA with a Masters in Nursing then went on to study nutritional science, functional medicine, quantum physics, genetics, neuro-immune-endocrinology, and metaphysical healing.

After working in a variety of traditional clinical settings for 10 years, she opened a solo private practice where she specializes in natural therapies. Through her extensive clinical research and two decades of collecting empirical data, Deborah developed a unique holistic health care model that blends naturopathic and allopathic therapies.

She also created a successful nutraceutical product called Genesis Gold®. This groundbreaking, holistic nutritional supplement, combined with her knowledge of natural healing therapies, has garnered Deborah widespread acclaim.

Deborah is the Founder of Full Circle Family Health, Genesis Health Products, Inc and Divine Daughters Unite - a nonprofit organization that benefits women. She serves as clinical endocrine advisor to Genova Laboratory and Sansum Medical Clinic, and she is also the past president of the California Association of Nurse Practitioners.

Author of the book, Hormones in Harmony®, and much-sought-after speaker, Deborah has given presentations at numerous professional and public events. Her list of speaking credits includes, the California Women's Expo, the Southern California Women's Herbal Symposium, Samuel Merritt College, and the American College of Nurse Practitioners.

Deborah resides in beautiful Ojai, California with her husband.

Made in the USA
Middletown, DE
03 May 2022